PENGUIN BOOKS

POOH'S WORKOUT BOOK

Ethan Mordden was educated at Friends
Academy and the University of Pennsylva-
nia, and has taught at Yale. He is the author
of twelve books, most recently *Demented:
The World of the Opera Diva*.

ALSO BY THE AUTHOR

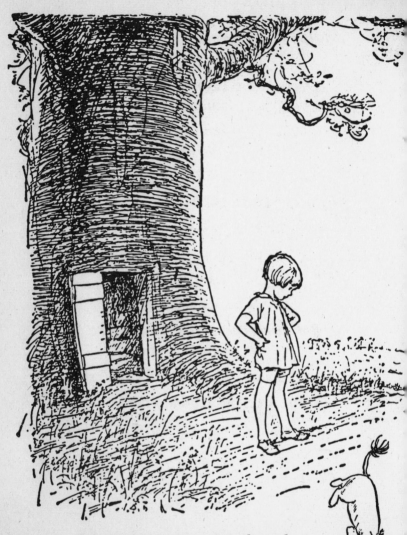

Illustrations by Ernest H. Shepard

Ethan Mordden

POOH'S
WORKOUT
BOOK

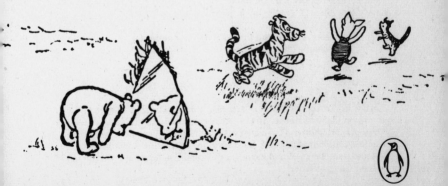

PENGUIN BOOKS

PENGUIN BOOKS

Viking Penguin Inc., 40 West 23rd Street, New York, New York 10010, U.S.A.
Penguin Books Ltd, Harmondsworth, Middlesex, England
Penguin Books Australia Ltd, Ringwood,
Victoria, Australia
Penguin Books Canada Limited, 2801 John Street,
Markham, Ontario, Canada L3R 1B4
Penguin Books (N.Z.) Ltd, 182–190 Wairau Road,
Auckland 10, New Zealand

First published in the United States of America by
E. P. Dutton, Inc., 1984
Published in Penguin Books 1985

Grateful acknowledgment is made to The Trustees of the Pooh Properties
for the use of illustrations by E. H. Shepard and quoted material
by A. A. Milne.
Individual copyrights for text quotations and illustrations: *When We
Were Very Young*, copyright 1924 by E. P. Dutton & Co., Inc.;
copyright renewal 1952 by A. A. Milne; *Winnie-the-Pooh*,
copyright 1926 by E. P. Dutton & Co., Inc.; copyright renewal 1953
by A. A. Milne; *Now We Are Six*, copyright 1927
by E. P. Dutton & Co., Inc.;
copyright renewal 1955 by A. A. Milne; *The House at Pooh Corner*,
copyright 1928 by E. P. Dutton & Co., Inc.; copyright renewal 1956
by A. A. Milne.

Printed in the United States of America by
R. R. Donnelley & Sons Company, Harrisonburg, Virginia.
Set in Caledonia

To my own forest creatures:
Scott and Lisa
Martha and David
Amy and Lauren
and Baby Watson

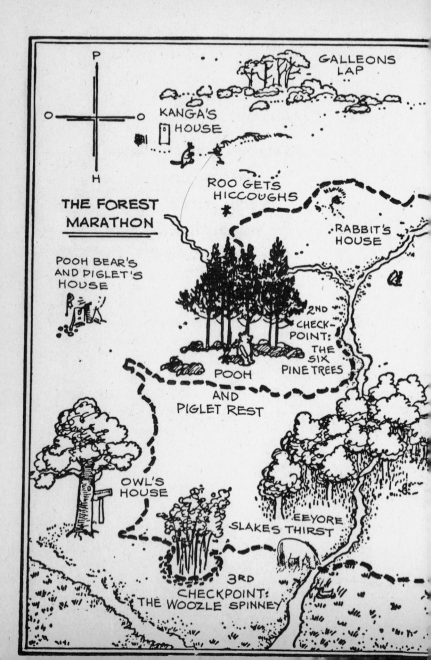

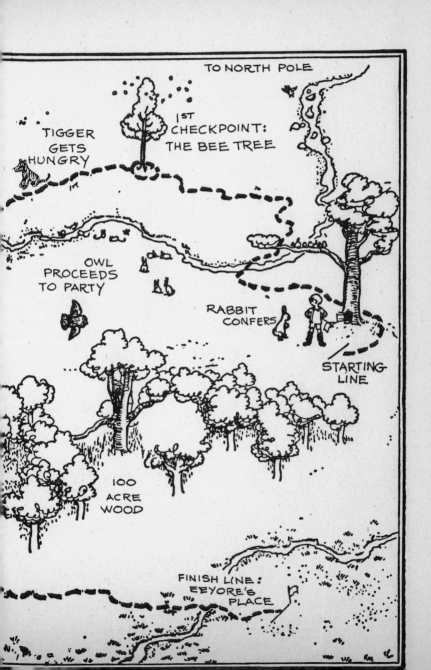

A bear, however hard he tries,
Grows tubby without exercise . . .

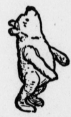

CONTENTS

ACKNOWLEDGMENT

The author wishes to acknowledge the collaboration of his editor, Jerret Engle, as being more than professional support and guidance. This time it truly was a collaboration: stimulating, original, and imaginative. Half this book is hers.

POOH'S
WORKOUT
BOOK

INTRODUCTION

"Pooh," I said one day when we were out walking with Piglet to nowhere in particular. "Exercise is the thing. You want to be fit. You want to tone up your muscles and stride through the Forest like a Bear of Great Strength."

"I do?" he said.

"Well, don't you?"

He wondered. "I haven't given it much thought."

"How about you, Piglet?" I went on. "Wouldn't you like to try looking at the world from a more self-confident angle? Just think—then you wouldn't have to worry about getting bounced by Tigger."

"I don't worry anymore," he answered.

"When I see Tigger coming, I get behind Pooh."

"Exercise," I persisted, "is the mode of the day. Everyone is taking it up—swimming, lifting weights, running, dancing . . ."

"I do my Stoutness Exercises," said Pooh. "Every morning. I stretch my arms up as high as they go and then I bend over and touch my toes with them."

"That's the spirit, Pooh!"

"At least, I *try* to touch my toes. Sometimes they're right there and sometimes they get out of reach. You never can tell with toes."

"How many sets do you do, and how many reps?"

"Sets?"

"How many times do you do it?"

"Oh, as many times as I can."

"Right. You've got to push yourself. What's your record so far?"

"Almost."

"Almost what?"

"I mean I've almost done it."

"*Once?* Your record for toe-touching is *almost once?*"

"Is that bad?"

"It's a somewhat skimpy showing for a daily exercise." Then, to cheer him up, I added, "But at least you're on the right track, starting the morning off with a calisthenic warmup." He did cheer up. "Now, what do you do after your toe-touchings?"

"I usually go to the cupboard to see about A Little Something."

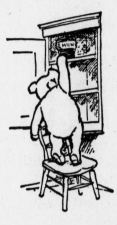

"No, no. I mean, then what *exercises* do you do?"

"You mean I'm supposed to do other ones?"

"That's the trouble with the Forest," I told him. "And it's not just you, Pooh. Everyone around here is cultivating a very lazy life. Piglet, do you do Stoutness Exercises like Pooh?"

"But I'm not stout," Piglet quickly pointed out.

"Exercise isn't just a remedy: it's also a deterrent. If you don't exercise, maybe you'll become stout."

"I think I *do* exercise," he replied. "Mine are different from Pooh's, that's all."

"Well, now we're getting somewhere. What's your favorite exercise? Jogging? Acrobatics?"

"Blowing dandelions."

"Piglet, that's *not* an exercise!"

"It is to the dandelions. I blow on the fluttery bits and they fly all about me through the air."

"Oh, for heaven's sake."

"I believe the fluttery bits are called dandies. At least, I hope they are."

I didn't speak again until we had passed through the Hundred Acre Wood and were just coming out into daylight again.

"What the Forest needs," I announced, "is a solid fitness program, a workout varied enough so that everyone can take part and can specialize in the exercises he finds most congenial. What do you say to that, Pooh?"

"How would that affect my Stoutness Exercise?"

"Well, for starters, you'd be able to do more than almost one."

"Would I have to give up blowing dandelions?" asked Piglet.

"You wouldn't have to give up anything, Piglet. You'd be getting, not losing."

"What would I get?"

"I'd like more birthdays," said Pooh.

"I'd like my very own haycorn tree," said Piglet, excited at the prospect. "And when all the haycorns have fallen off, I would hang balloons on it—"

"Yes! And how would you get up into the tree to hang the balloons?" I asked him, cleverly steering us back to the hard fact of exercise.

"I forgot about the climbing part," he finally answered.

"I could climb up for you, Piglet," said Pooh. "Bears are good at climbing trees."

"Thank you, Pooh."

"But then, of course," he added sadly, "there's always the getting-back-down part."

"I know a way," I said, "by which you, Piglet, could learn to climb trees and hang balloons—and you, Pooh, could master getting back down."

"How?" they both asked.

"Exercise!"

They said nothing, though I caught them sharing a Doubtful Look.

By this time, we had reached Eeyore's damp and gloomy corner of the Forest.

"Hallo, Eeyore!" we all cried.

He greeted us a little coolly, keeping an eye on

a patch of thistles, as if trying to decide if he should eat it right then despite a Social Call or save it for later.

"Eeyore," I began, "let me ask you a question. When you wake up of a morning—let's say on one of those brilliantly bright sunny days when it seems as though the whole world were smiling down on you in particular—what's the first activity that comes to mind?"

"Predicting rain," he replied.

"Rain?"

"Sometimes an earthquake. Why do you ask?"

"Actually, I was hoping that you would tell me about some favorite early-morning exercise."

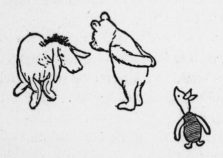

"Predicting rain is an exercise."

I sighed.

"I have to look up, don't I? To examine the sky? I have to crane my neck, do I not, so as not to miss any Menacing Clouds? You two-legged creatures don't realize how hard it is to gaze upward from a lower vantage point. But don't mind me. It's only four-legged Eeyore. Leave me out of your next party, that's all right. My neck will probably be so stiff from looking up that I wouldn't be able to come anyway." He eyed his thistle patch meaningfully.

"I'm sorry, Eeyore. Maybe you're right. I suppose that in looking upward you do develop the trapezius muscles."

"Develop the what?"

"The muscles in the neck and upper middle of the back. Predicting rain is probably very good for them."

"Very bad for them, too," he noted. "Overworks them. Then they hurt. And where's the fun in that, I ask you? Think about how others feel, next time you want to rhapsodize about their neck muscles."

"I'm sorry, Eeyore, really. I didn't—"

"That's right. Song and dance. Fa-la-ra. Here today and away tomorrow, without so much as a 'How is our trapezius holding up, Eeyore?' or 'Will a mustard plaster help, Eeyore?'"

Noticing that Eeyore was staring ever more

intently at his thistle patch, I hastily excused myself and moved on to canvass the Forest for any possible encouragement in the institution of a serious exercise program.

However, it was the same story, more or less, everywhere I went. Owl simply talked his way around the subject, using words like Stereopticon and Practicality, and alluding to an experience of his great-uncle once removed, involving a punting pole. Tigger and Roo were very unfocused. Kanga only said, "We'll see."

"Organization," Rabbit told me, "is what's needed. Teams and competitions. Pooh and Piglet and the rest are all right in their way, but they don't have Spirit. They have to be Told What to Do."

I said Thank you and headed on to Christopher Robin's house. He had spent the morning trying to figure out twice thirty-seven and three times eleven, and was very receptive to the idea of Getting Out and Doing Something.

"We could have another Expotition," he suggested. "Perhaps we ought to discover the South Pole this time. I don't believe anyone has yet. They hadn't up to yesterday."

"Well, actually—"

"Or we could go on a picnic!"

"What I had in mind was something more . . . well, more Exercisish."

"Oh, of course," he said. He said it carelessly, but he was looking at me the way he sometimes looks at Owl.

"I mean," I quickly added, "something more in the line of the usual workout routine, with some running, some pushups, and—"

"Pooh!"

"What?"

"And Piglet!"

"Hallo, Christopher Robin!" they cried, as they came up the hill.

"I've just been telling Christopher Robin about the Forest's new workout program," I interjected, after they had hugged each other. "I thought we would set up a Schedule so everyone can develop at his own speed in his own way, using the exercises that he prefers."

"Like blowing dandelions?" asked Piglet.

"And climbing trees?" asked Pooh. "Especially hunny trees?"

"Then we could all play Poohsticks!" cried Christopher Robin.

"There's a new dandelion patch over by the Woozle trees," said Piglet. "It called out to me as I passed it yesterday, and I promised to come as soon as I could. I expect I might bring a few friends."

"Let's go there now," said Christopher Robin.

It isn't precisely my idea of a stimulating af-

ternoon, but I went along, to keep in touch with
Local Habits until I could develop an approach to
the Considerable Problem of Bringing Exercise to
the Forest.

1. PLANNING
A FITNESS PROGRAM

"Some are thin and nimble, some pudgy and a bit slow, and some strong and fast," I said, "and that's the way it is. Different exercises for different shapes. That's what I call a fitness routine."

"Which am I?" Pooh asked.

"I'm thin," said Piglet.

"I'm strong," said Tigger.

Everyone looked at Pooh.

"Am I pudgy?" he asked.

"Pooh," I said, "we all have to pursue exercise in our individual way. And I'm willing to work with everyone on an individualized basis. Piglet can specialize in his thin and nimble exercises, Tigger in his strong and fast ones. And you, Pooh—"

"Can specialize in Pudgy and a Bit Slow Exercises?" He seemed crushed.

"Why not think of them as exercises for the Pooh Shape?" I said.

"The Pooh Shape?" He looked intrigued at being a Source of Classification.

"I mean," I went on, "that exercise should fit the individual, instead of the individual having to fit the exercise."

"Like a bear eats hunny," Pooh suggested, "but hunny doesn't eat a bear?"

"Somewhat."

"Well, what fits a Bear of . . . what was it you said yesterday?"

"A Bear of Great Strength?"

"A Bear of Great Strength-to-Be," Pooh amended, "formerly Pudgy. What exercise should I try?"

"There's no should about it, Pooh. What exercise would you *like* to try?"

"Do I know any? I mean, the kind you like?"

"You know a great many, though you may not think of them as exercises." I turned to the others. "All of you have been exercising right along," I said. "You've just been going about it unsystematically and in unusual ways. For instance you, Pooh, are always climbing trees and digging Heffalump traps. I'll admit it's a somewhat out-of-the-way sport, but it is a sound calisthenic. Tigger, you almost never stop moving. If we could only channel that energy into a fitness routine! And Piglet, you've had many a brush with athletics just through proximity to Pooh."

"Are there other Shapes?" Piglet asked. "That have exercises?"

"As a matter of fact, there's the Piglet Shape."

His nose wrinkled in thought. "The thin and nimble one?"

"Exactly. And lastly, there's the Tigger Shape, strong and . . ."

Tigger was so appreciative of being a Shape that he did three somersaults and two back flips, chased his tail around a gorse-bush, and came crashing back to end up, somehow, sitting in several places at once.

". . . and fast," I concluded, helping Piglet up. "But let's try to hold off exercising, everyone, till we can work out the appropriate techniques, timings, and—"

"—location," Piglet suggested, eyeing Tigger from behind Pooh.

"If Piglet is thin and nimble," said Pooh, "and Tigger is strong and fast, that leaves only pudgy and a bit slow. Is that what I am, then?"

"Now, don't lose heart, Pooh. Let's take a reading of the three shapes one at a time, so we can differentiate each one's features. That way we may set certain goals and choose our individual exercises around them. Let's take the Pooh Shape first."

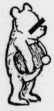

As our anonymous model reveals, the Pooh Shape tends to a rounded, thick trunk, with heavy limbs and very little neck.

STRENGTHS: lovability and loyalty.

WEAKNESS: Very Little Brain.

DIET PROBLEMS: over-emphasis on honey and condensed milk; too few green vegetables and fiber.

"Right away, certain measures are indicated: flexibility exercises, a lot of stretch-and-flex, weight-loss drills—"

"Is there a shape for Heffalumps, too?"

"Not now, Piglet, I'm demonstrating. And,

Pooh, I think we may want to try you out on some advanced gymnastics."

"All right," he replied. "As long as I'm back home for my elevenses. I generally like to take a little something round about then."

"I'll come with you, Pooh," said Piglet. "I expect it's just about eleven right now."

"Stay right where you are, everybody! Piglet, let's try your Shape now."

The Piglet Shape tends to a lean, compact body mass, with supple limbs, and a great deal of neck.

STRENGTHS: good intentions.

WEAKNESSES: lack of power and poor attitude.

DIET PROBLEMS: emphasis on haycorns shows over-reliance on macrobiotic nutrition.

"Piglet, what you need is to get out there and do it. You need to think rugged. Think *tough!*"

"It's eleven o'clock, Pooh. Shouldn't we—"
"Hold it right there. Tigger, you're next."

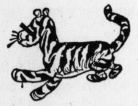

The Tigger Shape is that of the natural athlete, well-muscled and coordinated for sport.

STRENGTHS: plenty.

WEAKNESS: lack of composure.

DIET PROBLEMS: None. Exclusive diet of Extract of Malt suggests phenomenal possibilities for development of infant tonic as athletic supplement.

"Well," I said, "that about covers it. Of course, if you don't watch your intake of Calories, you're going to deprive your Shape of its Definition."

"What are Calories?" Pooh asked.

"Calories are honey, condensed milk, and birthday cake."

"Everything Pooh likes best," Piglet whispered.

"Haycorns, too," I added.

"Piglet's favorite," said Pooh, awed.

"Actually, Calories are everything—if you have too much of it. Fitness takes in more than calisthenics, you know. It's a matter of getting essential nutrients and watching those little smackerels of something."

"Watch them do what?" Pooh asked.

"I don't mean 'look at them,' Pooh—I mean count them. Too many smackerels can change your Shape. You remember what happened that time at Rabbit's!"

Pooh always liked a little something at eleven o'clock in the morning, and he was very glad to see Rabbit getting out the plates and mugs; and when Rabbit said, "Honey or condensed milk with your bread?" he was so excited that he said, "Both," and then, so as not to seem greedy, he added, "But don't bother about the bread, please." And for a long time after that he said nothing . . . until at last, humming to himself in a rather sticky voice, he got up, shook Rabbit lovingly by the paw, and said that he must be going on.

So he started to climb out of the hole. He pulled with his front paws, and pushed with his back paws, and in a little while his nose was out in the open again . . . and then his ears . . . and then his front paws . . . and then his shoulders . . . and then—

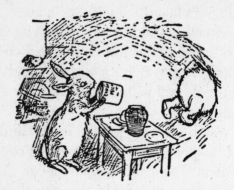

"Oh, help!" said Pooh. "I'd better go back."

"Oh, bother!" said Pooh. "I shall have to go on."

"I can't do either!" said Pooh. "Oh, help *and* bother!"

Now by this time Rabbit wanted to go for a walk too, and finding the front door full, he went out by the back door, and came round to Pooh, and looked at him.

"Hallo, are you stuck?" he asked.

"N-no," said Pooh carelessly. "Just resting and thinking and humming to myself."

"Here, give us a paw."

Pooh Bear stretched out a paw, and Rabbit pulled and pulled and pulled . . .

"It all comes," said Pooh crossly, "of not having front doors big enough."

"It all comes," said Rabbit sternly, "of eating too much. I thought at the time," said Rabbit, "only I didn't like to say anything," said Rabbit, "that one of us was eating too much," said Rabbit, "and I knew it wasn't *me*," he said.

"Did Calories do that?" asked Tigger.

"No," Piglet said. "Pooh did that."

"By taking in too many Calories!" I added triumphantly. "There now, Pooh, don't you see?"

"Next time I'll go out the back door," Pooh vowed.

"Why not simply have a smaller smackerel?"

Pooh looked worried. "That might mean stopping by Rabbit's a bit more often."

"*No*, Pooh. That might mean keeping your Shape in trim! And you do that by *skipping* those extra smackerels."

"How do I know which ones are extra?"

"You still haven't told us," Piglet cried, "if there's a Heffalump Shape!"

"Piglet, there is no such thing as a Heffalump. I'm sorry, but we must be scientific. If we get off on the wrong foot, there's no telling—"

"No such thing as Heffalumps?" Pooh echoed.

"I just *saw* one yesterday," cried Tigger.

"You saw a Heffalump?" I asked him. "That's impossible."

Tigger growled.

"Maybe it was something else," Piglet suggested nervously. "A Woozle, perhaps?"

"All right, everyone, let's break for today. Tomorrow we'll try out a few beginner's exercises."

Pooh and Piglet went off hand in hand, and Tigger romped away. "This is not going to be easy," I thought to myself.

2. EXERCISES FOR
THE TIGGER SHAPE

"Tigger," I began, when we were all assembled at our meeting place near the Six Pine Trees, "as you are the Forest's most constant athlete, why don't you lead off the session?"

"All right."

"I've explained that exercise works best when it is geared to the individual—to his Shape and his personal taste. Now, Tigger, you have a distinctive and very individual exercise. It's simple, good for just about every part of the body, requires no props, and can be done anywhere. Why don't you tell us about it?"

We all looked at Tigger expectantly.

Tigger smiled nervously.

We all looked a little more expectantly.

Tigger grinned nervously.

So we all looked at Tigger with Extreme Expectation (and a little impatience), and he backed away a bit and said, "Tell you about what?"

"You know . . . that famous . . . oh, you know, that jitter with a sort of dashing push in it and a touch of crash. *You* know."

"He means Tigger's *bouncing*," said Piglet, getting behind Pooh.

"Shh," Tigger told me. "Don't let the others hear."

"It's a little late to keep it a secret. Besides, **Bouncing** is a fine exercise, and a very Friendly one."

"That," said Piglet, "depends on who is doing the bouncing."

BOUNCING

TECHNIQUE

Strangely, there are very little data on this celebrated exercise. No manual you might consult shows anything in the way of procedural exposition or diagram. In fact, the manuals scarcely mention bouncing at all.

How does one bounce, then? How *exactly*? This is like asking, How does water get wet? You

don't ask, you just bounce. And *how* you bounce is
. . . well, as Tigger explained it, "I just see someone
I know, and that makes me feel Friendly, so I sort of
patter up near him to say something or so."

"He comes up *behind*," said Piglet. "And fast!"

"No, I don't. I come up near his back for a
Friendly Surprise. And then I sort of . . . I . . ."

"Bungle all over him," Piglet filled in. "Why
don't you ask Tigger to tell about the Hazards of
Bouncing?"

HAZARDS OF BOUNCING

Well, there are hazards in any sport, and I
must admit bouncing is somewhat controversial,
though nowhere near as much so nowadays as it
was when Tigger first arrived in the Forest with his
habit of Bouncing by Friendly Surprise. (See Diagram A.)

"How did you fall in, Eeyore?" asked Rabbit.

"I didn't," said Eeyore.

"But how—"

"I was BOUNCED," said Eeyore.

"Oo," said Roo excitedly, "did somebody push
you?"

"Somebody BOUNCED me. I was just thinking by
the side of the river—thinking, if any of you know

what that means—when I received a loud
BOUNCE."

"Oh, Eeyore!" said everybody.

"Are you sure you didn't slip?" asked Rabbit
wisely.

"Of course I slipped. If you're standing on the slip-
pery bank of a river, and somebody BOUNCES you
loudly from behind, you slip. What did you think I
did?"

"But who did it?"

Eeyore didn't answer.

"I expect it was Tigger," said Piglet nervously.

"You bounced me," said Eeyore to Tigger gruffly.

"I didn't really. I had a cough, and I happened to
be behind Eeyore, and I said *'Grrrr-oppp-
ptschschschz.'*"

This last remark is a fair if somewhat sketchy
description of how bouncing is performed, hazard-
ous though it be.

Experts have not been able to agree on
whether it is more beneficial to give a bounce than
to receive it, but the Forest has agreed that Tigger
had best concentrate on bouncing only at those
who like getting bounced, such as Tigger's shadow,
which puts up with it, and Roo, who entirely enjoys

DIAGRAM A: A TYPICAL BOUNCING HAZARD

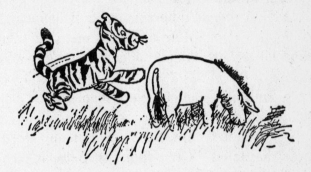

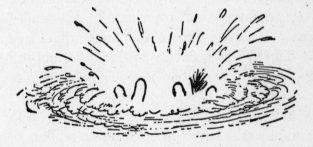

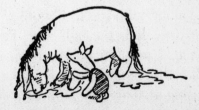

it. Beginners who wish to attempt it might want to get into open country first, so as not to risk any Bouncing Hazards. (See Diagram A again.)

"I don't think I'd be very good at bouncing," says Pooh. "Even after all the time I've spent around Tigger, I still don't understand exactly what bouncing is for."

"I don't like bouncing very much at *all*," said Piglet.

Tigger didn't reply to this in so many words, but he muttered *"Grrrr-oppp-ptschschschz"* and stalked off.

"I'm not giving up on you yet, Piglet," I went on. "I can understand your fear of bouncing— bouncing is really far more adapted to the Tigger Shape than to yours. But I've got another possibility, an exercise as lively as bouncing but much less intimidating."

"I'll listen," said Piglet, but he looked as if I'd just told him that haycorns grow on umbrellas.

"I could use another exercise myself," said Pooh. "I don't have even one yet."

"Come along with me to Eeyore's," I said.

As we traveled through the Forest at a Friendly pace, I pointed out to Pooh and Piglet that, whether they knew it or not, all three of us were exercising at that very moment. "Walking is one of the handiest exercises of all," I said. "It's fun and it's useful."

"I like walking because I like to walk," said Piglet, "not because it's an exercise."

"If walking is a good exercise," said Pooh, "how come I'm pudgy? Yesterday I walked to the North Pole."

"Why, Pooh?" asked Piglet.

"To see if it was in the same place as when I discovered it." He turned to me. "If I walked all the way to the North Pole and back, I should be a Bear of Great Strength already. Shouldn't I?"

"No, Pooh, and that's just my point. To get anything out of your exercising, you have to program it into a Daily Routine."

"You mean walk to the North Pole every day?"

"I mean exercise every day. The same exercises, in the same order. And *then* you'll be a Bear of Great Strength."

"I thought exercise was like a party," said Piglet. "Where you have it and then it's over."

"No, Piglet. It's never over."

"You mean exercise is . . ."

"Forever."

It was one of those afternoons when it doesn't much matter if you went and did something just now or a year from next Thursday. I could see my two companions watching the brooks and streams as we passed them and they passed us, watched them listen for birdsong and dote on the shades of green, brown, yellow, and red that the Forest was wearing. Nothing was further from their thoughts than the advantages of a sound fitness routine.

Nor was Eeyore in an assistant mood. "Here they come again," he observed as we called out our hallos. "Running and jumping and falling down, and when they pick themselves up they stop and say, 'Why don't we go down and get Eeyore to strain his neck muscles for us? That should be fun.'" He snorted, turned sideways, stamped his hooves, and snorted again. "This is what comes of fluff in the head instead of brains."

"Actually, Eeyore," I began, "we have come to you to get some advice on a field in which you are the expert. You and you alone."

"No, I'm not," he sniffed. "What field?"

"The Field of Positive Frisking, of course. Don't you remember the day you introduced **The Frisk**? When you lost your tail? Pooh happened to pay a call on Owl, who had just hung up a new doorbell:

"Handsome bell-rope, isn't it?" said Owl.

Pooh nodded.

"It reminds me of something," he said, "but I can't think what. Where did you get it?"

"I just came across it in the Forest. It was hanging over a bush, and I thought at first somebody lived there, so I rang it, and nothing happened, and then I rang it again very loudly, and it came off in my hand, and as nobody seemed to want it, I took it home, and—"

"Owl," said Pooh solemnly, "you made a mistake. Somebody did want it."

"Who?"

"Eeyore. My dear friend Eeyore. He was—he was fond of it."

"Fond of it?"

"Attached to it," said Winnie-the-Pooh sadly.

"I distinctly remember how happy you were," I went on to Eeyore, "when Christopher Robin nailed it back on for you."

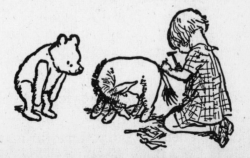

"Expansive fellow, that Owl," Eeyore re-marked. "Very generous with other people's things. A tail may seem worthless to you, but it has its charms."

"You could scarcely do the frisk without it. However, some athletes may want to try, so let us go through it step by step."

FRISKING

"First, bracing yourself sturdily against the earth, lower your head all the way down, almost to the ground. Then push it a little farther to look behind you. This will toughen the neck muscles, by the way."

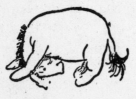

Step 1.

"There you go," Eeyore moaned, "with the neck muscles again."

"As you look behind you, you may or may not see a waggly tail-like thing, which, if you *do* see it, you should immediately and enthusiastically admire."

"What if they don't see it?"

"Then they should pretend they do, since Tail Admiration is an integral part of the frisk."

"Maybe Christopher Robin could tack one on for them," Pooh suggested.

"Strictly for frisk purposes," Eeyore put in. "They'll have to bring it back directly after."

"Now for the second step: flip around to face in the opposite direction, stand straight and tall—"

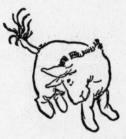

Step 2.

"And they'll bump their heads on a low-lying branch of a hostile tree."

"—and, curving the head to the side, fondly gaze upon, while merrily wagging, the tail."

"You should remember to tell them that the frisk should be reserved only for times when A Glad

Surprise Changes the Tone of One's Life. That will save them a lot of trouble, as it doesn't happen often. Almost never, in fact."

"Well, Eeyore, perhaps the frisk should be maintained as an everyday exercise, to function as its own glad surprise for a sunny day."

"Don't mind me. Go right ahead. Run a good thing into the ground."

"*In step three*—if everyone is listening, thank you very much—in step three, you sit back on your hindquarters and muse more or less deliriously upon the tail from above."

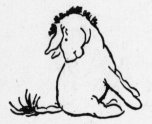

Step 3.

"And what if they should fall over backwards and crush the tail? 'Think about tomorrow, you who frolic thoughtlessly today': that's *my* advice."

"And lastly, for step four: leap forward to balance on your head with the rest of the body piled on top, kick the rear legs in bicycle fashion, flop the tail around as merrily as it will flop, and bray with uncontrollable delight.

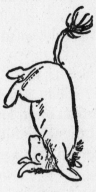

Step 4.

"Have you anything to add to that, Eeyore? Being the presiding master of the frisk and all?"

He looked away pensively, then said, "Pooh, did you really call me your 'dear friend Eeyore'?"

Now Pooh looked away, so Piglet spoke up: "Yes, Eeyore, I believe he did."

Eeyore considered this, then said, "He must have been thinking of someone else."

APPLIED FRISKING

We had settled on an exercise that had a lot of potential, I thought, for general Forest use. Sometime later, when we were alone at the Six Pine Trees, I attempted coaching Pooh in the art of frisking.

"I suppose I could try it," he said, "just after working on a Hum."

"Exactly. What would make a day Hummier than a good frisk?"

"You don't think the frisk is wrong for the Pooh shape? I mean, would it feel quite as . . . as frisky on two legs instead of on four?"

"Hmm. I hadn't thought of it that way."

"Then there's the tail part. I'm not sure I could admire mine as easily as Eeyore can admire his. Of course, I've got a tail. I can feel it tailing behind me. I just don't see it very often."

"Well, let's forget about the tail part. Try frisking for the fun of it. After all, Pooh, fun is the main thing in a frisk. The tail part is optional."

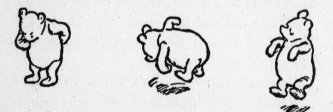

Pooh tried frisking. I must say, he really did throw himself into it. I called out the instructions for each step, and he did his best. But he couldn't help looking for his tail—and, it's true, Pooh's tail somehow never gets into an angle appropriate for Admiration.

I thought it crucial not to get bogged down in failure at this stage, but neither did I want to encourage Pooh in the tempting art of Quitting. So I left Pooh to practice—with a few words of encouragement—and moved onward to see about propagating the frisk among the other Forest creatures. The frisk, I felt, had the attractions of a genuine breakthrough exercise: it's easy, it's healthful, and it's silly. How could it miss?

Indeed, though Kanga thought she got quite enough exercise leaping through the Forest with Roo in her pocket and Tigger bouncing along behind her, Roo and Tigger themselves took to frisking with abandon. They even developed variations on frisk procedures, Roo in the assimilation of what he called "the splunk," an added finale in which the friskee leaps up to fall flat on his back in the sandy pit crying out "Splunk!"

"It needs more height," Rabbit noted, as he passed on his way to consult with Owl. Christopher Robin was out when I dropped by, but I felt sure he would want to sample the frisk, and perhaps reinvent it in a version for himself and Pooh. Feeling quite content about the way things were shaping up, I came upon Pooh still trying the frisk where I had left him. He seemed dejected.

"It isn't working," he told me.

"Never mind, Pooh. There are plenty of exercises where that one came from."

"Is it because I'm pudgy and a bit slow?"

"I'll tell you what—tomorrow we'll try some special exercises for the Pooh Shape!"

He brightened up somewhat. "I have a Hum about The Pleasures of the Pooh Shape. Would you like to hear it?"

"Of course."

And he sang it:

> *I could spend a happy morning*
> > *Seeing Roo,*
> *I could spend a happy morning*
> > *Being Pooh.*
> *For it doesn't seem to matter*
> *If I don't get any fatter*
> *(And I don't get any fatter)*
> > *What I do.*

"It's one of my best," he said.

"A classic, Pooh. But the problem is, you *do* get fatter. And stuck in Rabbit's front door."

"I'd forgotten about that."

"I have an idea. Why don't you make up a *new* Hum About the Pleasures of the Pooh Shape? One that knows about the hazards of smackerels. You could sing it to yourself whenever you do your Daily Routine!"

It was devious of me, perhaps, but it seemed a reasonable way to interest Pooh in his athletic progress.

"A new Hum! Of course! And then tomorrow I can teach my new Pooh Shape Hum to everyone and we won't have to bother about exercises!"

"Well . . . no, Pooh. Why don't you exercise and *then* sing your Hum?"

"Oh, all right." And off he went, working on a Hum. I wondered if I might try running an aerobics class to the Hums of Pooh.

Well, it's a thought.

3. EXERCISES FOR
THE POOH SHAPE

"My new Hum on 'The Pleasures of the Pooh Shape' is all ready," Pooh announced. "I mean, I'm willing to sing it, if someone should by any chance want to hear it."

"Of course we want to hear it," said Christopher Robin.

"I'd like to hear it twice," said Piglet. "Then I'd like to go home and pick some haycorns."

"We're all here," I said, perhaps a little loudly, "to discuss some exercises especially designed for the Pooh Shape. Now, Pooh, how would you like to start?"

"I'd like to start by singing my Hum."

The others cheered.

"I meant, what exercise would you like to start with?"

He looked perplexed. "But I don't know any."

"Sure you do. What happens when you see a tempting beehive up in a tree?"

"I might climb up to look at the hunny. Just to see if it's all right."

"There you are. That's your exercise: climbing a tree."

"Then he might fall out of the tree," said Piglet. "Is that part of the exercise?"

"Maybe it should be," said Pooh.

"Pooh, falling out of a tree is not an exercise."

"Oh. Well, what is it, then?"

"It's . . . well, it's . . . it doesn't matter what it is. It matters what it isn't. And it *isn't* exercise."

"Didn't you say we could plan our own exercises?" said Piglet. "Why can't Pooh plan **Falling Out of Trees**?"

Pooh appealed to Christopher Robin. "Isn't falling an exercise?"

"It all depends," Christopher Robin replied, patting Pooh on the head. "Sometimes it is and sometimes it isn't."

"Couldn't we just try it?" Pooh asked me. "Just to see?"

FALLING OUT OF TREES

Granted, this is not a standard exercise for any

Shape. It is not only unorthodox; it might be revolutionary. But as some of the larger Forest creatures habitually climb trees only to find that they can't effectively climb *down*, I had to consider falling as a Forest activity, to be dealt with in terms of timing, technique, and form.

TIMING

Timing procedures in falling are still undeveloped in the Forest at the present writing. Local experts will debate the precise climatic and scenic conditions preparatory to a successful bouncing session, or compare addenda on the occasions that make for a truly satisfying frisk. At least, I hope they will. However, no one has as yet set a moment when it is right to fall out of a tree.

"A branch goes crack," Pooh explains, "and there you are."

"Or, rather, there you were."

Pooh nods. "It's the same thing."

TECHNIQUE

Should one fall loosely, with dangling limbs and a merry heart? Should one fall tightly, rolled up like something about to be wrapped in a Christmas box, trying to think of nothing, or of a very small slice of seedy cake? Here, too, research stands on the cursory side, perhaps because falling, when it does occur, is over rather quickly. The experiential data are lacking.

FORM

We can, at least, discuss form; indeed, I discussed it with both Pooh and Tigger, the Forest stalwarts in the sport. Let us compare Pooh's form with Tigger's. Pooh favors the nonchalant, head-down approach:

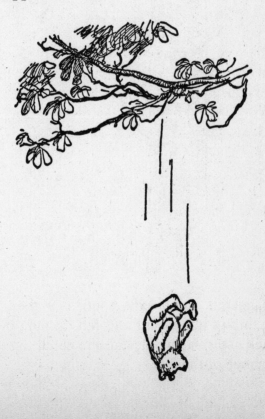

and breaks his fall by crashing into low-lying branches on his way down.

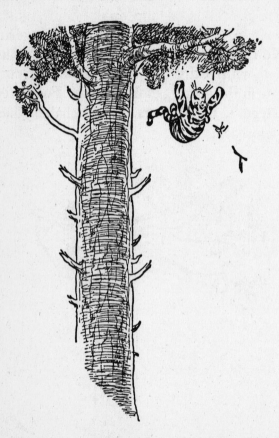

Tigger, a more agile sportsman than Pooh, really throws himself into his fall, turning over on his back and splaying his limbs to catch the simple exuberance of the feat.

One might say that Pooh falls in a lump, Tigger in a fling. Note, however, that where Pooh fin-
ishes off in the natural setting, on whatever is under
him, Tigger takes advantage of a ready cohort,
waiting to catch him in—as here—Christopher
Robin's tunic.

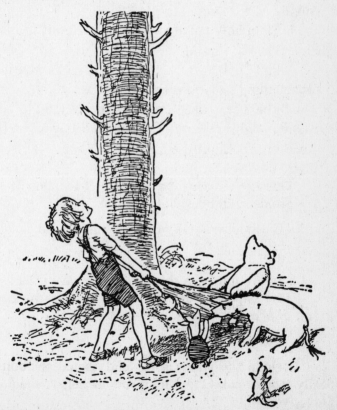

"What if you are not available," I asked Christopher Robin, "or find yourself under-equipped?"

He thought for a minute. "You could always use a sheet," he offered. "But my tunic works best."

"Well," I concluded, "it certainly looks like fun, leaping down through the sky to the waiting earth."

"Then how come you haven't tried it?" asked Piglet.

"Pooh," I hurriedly rejoined, "let's consider other falling situations that might arise."

"There was that time Pooh pretended to be a cloud!" Christopher Robin recalled eagerly. "Remember, Pooh? At the honey tree?"

One bee sat down on the nose of the cloud for a moment, and then got up again.

"Christopher—*ow!*—Robin," called out the cloud.

"Yes?"

"I have just been thinking, and I have come to a very important decision. *These are the wrong sort of bees.*"

"Are they?"

"Quite the wrong sort. So I should think they would make the wrong sort of honey, shouldn't you?"

"Would they?"

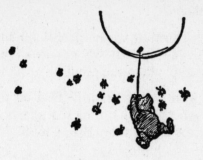

"Yes. So I think I shall come down."

"How?"

Winnie-the-Pooh hadn't thought about this. If he let go of the string he would fall—*bump*—and he didn't like the idea of that. So he thought for a long time, and then he said:

"Christopher Robin, you must shoot the balloon with your gun. Have you got your gun?"

"Of course I have. But if I do that, it will spoil the balloon."

"But if you *don't*," said Pooh, "I shall have to let go, and that would spoil *me*."

Christopher Robin aimed very carefully at the balloon, and fired.

"*Ow!*" said Pooh.

"Did I miss?"

"You didn't exactly *miss*," said Pooh, "but you missed the *balloon*."

"I'm so sorry." This time Christopher Robin hit the balloon, and the air came slowly out, and Winnie-the-Pooh floated down to the ground.

But his arms were so stiff from holding on to the string of the balloon all that time that they stayed up straight in the air for more than a week.

"And what about the time Pooh fell into the Heffa-lump trap?" cried Piglet. He looked at me. "I suppose you're going to tell me that there's no such thing as Heffalump traps."

I looked away and whistled.

"I guess I do fall a lot," said Pooh. "I don't try to, but I do, and there it is."

Pooh was so busy not looking where he was going that he stepped on a piece of the Forest which had been left out by mistake; and he only just had time to think to himself: "I'm flying. What Owl does. I wonder how you stop—" when he stopped.

Bump!

"Ow!" squeaked something.

"That's funny," thought Pooh. "I said 'Ow!' without really oo'ing."

"Help!" said a small, high voice.

"That's me again," thought Pooh. "I've had an Accident, and fallen down a well, and my voice has gone all squeaky and works before I'm ready for it, because I've done something to myself inside. Bother!"

"Help—help!"

"There you are! I say things when I'm not trying. So it must be a very bad Accident." And then he thought that perhaps when he did try to say things he wouldn't be able to; so, to make sure, he said loudly: "A Very Bad Accident to Pooh Bear."

"Pooh!" squeaked the voice.

"It's Piglet!" cried Pooh eagerly. "Where are you?"

"Underneath," said Piglet in an underneath sort of way.

"Underneath what?"

"You," squeaked Piglet. "Get up!"

"You *do* fall a lot, Pooh," I said. "Maybe we ought to devise a chart on it, to compare the right and wrong methods. Then newcomers to the sport could benefit from your expertise."

"They *could?*"

"See, Pooh?" said Christopher Robin.

"They may want to learn my Hum, too."

"Let's make our chart first," I said.

BOX ON FALLING, BY POOH

FALLING FROM A TREE:
Look where you're going.

WRONG RIGHT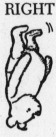

FALLING INTO A HEFFALUMP TRAP:
Land right side up.

WRONG RIGHT

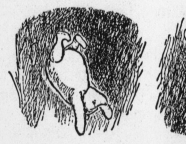

Pooh made this box.

THE TOUCHDOWN

"One thing we haven't accounted for yet, Pooh," I said, "is possible landing places for when you do fall."

"Yes, Pooh," Piglet agreed. "Then you won't have to fall on me."

"I never thought I'd have to arrange about that," he replied. "When I fall there's always been something hard under me, sooner or later."

"Why not land in something soft?"

"I'd like to," said Pooh. "If only someone would put out a great pile of leaves right where I'm falling, there would be much less Bother."

"What do you usually land in, Pooh?"

"I *seem* to prefer gorse-bushes, although I don't remember ever Making a Decision about it. They just always seem to be there when I fall."

"I don't like gorse-bushes," said Christopher Robin.

"Nor I," said Piglet. "Though of course I'm not as familiar with them as Pooh."

"The thing about gorse-bushes," said Pooh, "is the way they have of springing out at you. Especially when you can't defend yourself properly, having momentarily lost your balance."

"Let's chart this exercise as fully as possible, Pooh," I said, "so others can take it into their workout routines. Because it has the makings of a good resistance exercise."

"But the *other* thing about gorse-bushes is their prickles. If you fall on them, they decide to visit with you, whether you want them to or not."

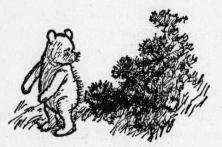

"This is where the resistance comes in, as the prickles bite you and you attempt to get away from them as quickly as possible. Perhaps this exercise should be called not Falling Into a Gorse-Bush but Jumping Quite Suddenly Out of One."

"Do I *have* to fall into a gorse-bush to exercise?" Pooh asked.

"Of course not. We're listing some general possibilities. Once we set them all down, we can choose the ones we prefer."

"I already don't prefer this one," Pooh observed. "It's not a good exercise for an animal who is likely to get Excitable in Discomfort."

"I should think this exercise really becomes most valuable in its resting-up-after period, from the concentration involved in pulling out the prickles, which probably get into all sorts of hard-to-reach places."

"That's the trouble with it," said Pooh. "You have to reach around the right way with the wrong hand, or the wrong way with the right hand. Gorse prickles never can be reached the right way with the right hand."

"I wonder why that is."

"Because," Christopher Robin put in, "gorse prickles are contrary."

"Well, anyway," I went on, "all that reaching and grabbing make for stretching motions to improve body tone and flexibility. So you see, Pooh," I added cleverly, "Jumping Quite Suddenly Out of a Gorse-Bush might be a real exercise after all!"

"In that case," Pooh rejoined, "I'd better sing my Hum now." And Pooh sang it:

> *Oh, a Pooh is not alone,*
> *For his Shape is all his own;*
> *And it wouldn't suit a lion*
> *Or a bee.*
>
> *The Shape and Pooh make two,*
> *For the Shape just fits the Pooh,*
> *And the Pooh just fits his Shape*
> *To a P.*

"Silly old bear," said Christopher Robin.

"Being 'On the Pleasures,' " said Pooh, " 'of the Pooh Shape.' "

"Delightful, Pooh," I said. "Now, how about a group frisk?"

"I can't," said Piglet, apologetically. "I promised Owl I'd watch him hang up a picture of his grandfather Solomon."

"I have to go to China," said Christopher Robin.

"I should sing Eeyore my new Hum," said Pooh.

I let them go. You can't force true exercise. But I liked to think I had scored a minor victory.

Attitude, I told myself. *Attitude.* That's how it begins.

4. EXERCISES FOR
THE PIGLET SHAPE

When launching a fitness program, you smaller creatures may be intimidated by the abundance of larger creatures, some of whom started larger, and some of whom simply got larger by beginning their workouts before you did.

"It's a little discouraging," Piglet explained, "when it looks as though you have the Piglet Shape while everyone else has the Tigger Shape."

To all those with the Piglet Shape, I say: Do not be daunted! Everybody has to start somewhere—and remember that you can adopt a program that will please your sense of well-being while it enhances your size. There's no need to take up bouncing just because the big animals do it; nor should you attempt the frisk if you're not in the mood. After all, who is planning your workout cycle? You or Tigger?

"You are planning it," Piglet said when we met for our session. "And I'm afraid of what might be in it."

"Wouldn't you like to be a Piglet of Great Strength?" I asked him.

He thought it over. "If I take up exercise," he said, "shouldn't I do the exercises I want to do? Wouldn't that be a nice Daily Routine?"

"I did say that exercise should accord with the individual, didn't I?"

"Could I plan my own exercises?"

"Of course."

"With Directions?"

"Why not?"

"Then I think I'm ready."

"At last! And what exercise will you try?"

"Blowing Dandelions. And could I tell about it myself?"

I sighed.

"And could I have a box for special instructions just like Pooh? Please?"

"All right, Piglet. But then I think we should discuss a more athletic exercise. Agreed?"

"Yes. Soon."

Anyway, here is his exercise, in his words:

"Blowing Dandelions is good for newcomers

because, while it's very daring, it doesn't need any
Bothersome warmup.

"First, find a dandelion patch and sit down in
its nicest part, where the sun is breathing most
sweetly. Then pluck a dandelion, but gently, so the
little dandies don't fall off.

"Holding the dandelion upright, think about
something nice, like how many candies you might
get at your next party. Then, leaning forward, blow
against the dandies.

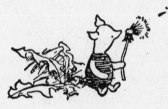

"You might blow hard and quickly, to scatter
the dandies in a great cluster all around you. You
might blow tenderly, as if telling the dandies how
your favorite candy tastes. You might blow them
way up high in a thin stream to dance on the wind,
or blow them into a tidy pile just next to you. My
favorite way is to blow on the dandies section by

section in a hush, so they fly for a bit, curve into a
fall, and lie there smiling at me. Is it time for my
box now?"

BLOWING DANDELIONS: CALORIES EXPENDED PER MINUTE, IN HAYCORNS

Blowing in a hush	8
Blowing hard and quickly	16
Blowing two dandelions at once	28
Blowing in a field frequented by Heffalumps	600

Box prepared by Piglet

"Very nice, Piglet," I had to say. "How do you
like exercise now?"

"It's all right," he answered.

"I always liked blowing on dandelions," said
Pooh, who had just joined us. "I never knew it was
good for the Pooh Shape. And other shapes, of
course."

"Well, now, Pooh, I wouldn't—"

"And just think, Pooh," said Piglet. "Whenever you exercise, you're allowed to celebrate with
a Little Extra Something."

"I hadn't thought of that," said Pooh. "Now I
like exercise. Every time I try frisking or Blowing
Dandelions, I'll go right home to replace the lost

smackerels. There's nothing worse for a Pooh Shape than a case of Hollow Tummy. Right?" he asked me.

"Pooh," I warned. "Exercise isn't an excuse to eat more. And as far as that goes, Piglet, blowing dandelions isn't much of a haycorn burner."

"You mean I have to do something else besides?" asked Piglet.

"Actually, I was rather hoping you would try the frisk today."

"I already have done. Before you came. I've been frisking for hours. Well, one hour, anyway. A few minutes. Once or twice."

"How did it go?"

"Quite well. I've decided to use it as my warmup exercise."

"Well, well. The Piglet Frisk."

"No. Mine is so different from Eeyore's that I've renamed it."

"Uh-oh."

"It's called **Jumping and Squeaking**."

"Piglet—"

"And I'm ready to share my discovery with other exercise victims, in my own words."

"Enthusiasts, Piglet, not victims. And I suppose you'll want a box again?"

"I might."

Anyway, here is Piglet's Jumping and Squeak-

ing. This time I am taking the lead in workout anal-
ysis—Piglet had to go make a little fir-cone house.

JUMPING AND SQUEAKING

TECHNIQUE

Jumping and Squeaking is an excellent way to
initiate your exercise hour, and has the added advantage of Creative Improvisation. Rather than follow some Bothering Routine, you jump and squeak
as the heart prompts and the mood of the day suggests. You can jump lightly (to limber up) or force-
fully (to work off Characteristic Anxieties of the
Piglet Shape). You can jump because the sun is
happy, or to defy the thunderclouds.

"Tell them they can make their jumping into a
How Long Can I Last?, to see how many jumps
they can take without stopping. Or they can jump
in groups separated by rest periods. And you left
out the squeaking. They can squeak while jumping,
in between each third jump, or after every group.
They can squeak any way they want, because this is
the perfect individual exercise, and ideally suited to
the Piglet Shape."

"If you say so yourself," I said. "Excuse me for
interrupting, but a How Long Can I Last? is called

an 'endurance event,' and it's not 'groups,' it's 'sets.' Sets and reps: the elements of exercise."

"There are no sets and reps in Jumping and Squeaking," said Piglet.

"Piglet, every exercise has sets and reps."

"Except mine."

VOLUME

The quality and amount of jumping and squeaking depends entirely on How You Feel Right Now, each creature's routine entirely different from all others. Piglet jumps sweetly, almost idyllically, as if trying to duplicate the motion of the earth. Christopher Robin works with a bit more enthusiasm. (See Figure A.)

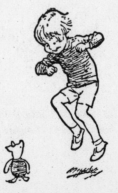

Figure A.

APPLICABILITY

Note that Piglet observes a low attitude so as not to lose his place when he comes down. Instead Piglet puts everything into his squeaking, in vigorous sessions that can go on for minutes, or until dessert.

"Now tell them that Roo's Jumping and Squeaking is disorganized. But this, too, is acceptable technique."

"Wait a minute!" I cried. "When did Roo take up Jumping and Squeaking?"

"I have to tell about the different styles, don't I?"

"But there aren't any yet."

"There will be. May I take over?"

I sighed heavily. He took over.

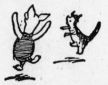

Jumping and Squeaking:
Two noted experts compare styles.

TIMING

"Roo doesn't even reserve a special time and place for jumping and squeaking, as Piglet (me) does, for the need of a Happy Release may come upon him at any moment.

"For some reason that I don't know, it most often comes upon him at bedtime, when he uses it as a ... oh, yes ... as an endurance event, to see how long he can keep it going. Unlike my jumping, Roo's moves all over the Forest. I call this 'traveling.' It may be a Bother, but it does keep the knees and toes nimble.

"No matter how exhausted Roo may be, he usually has a few good squeaks left for just before Kanga tucks him in. Also while she tucks him in. Also after."

PIGLET'S BOX

"Now I have to have my box, which shows how to Jump and Squeak."

"Piglet, you don't want a box; you want a diagram."

"All right, but I want to do it myself."

"As you wish."

"But will you help me?"

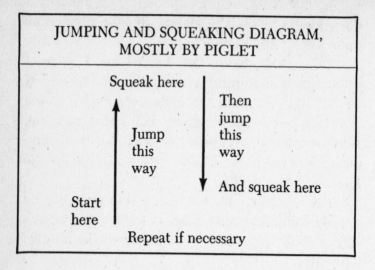

JUMPING AND SQUEAKING DIAGRAM,
MOSTLY BY PIGLET

Squeak here

Then
jump
this
way

Jump
this
way

And squeak here

Start
here

Repeat if necessary

CONCLUSION

Jumping and Squeaking especially suits the small body mass. Pooh finds it an unaccommodating activity, but then the springier sorts of exercise are hard on animals with the Pooh Shape.

"Does that mean I can't Jump and Squeak?" Pooh asked. He looked rather left out.

"Well, this one calls for someone thin and agile," I told him. "You remember what happened when you tried to frisk."

"I'm sorry, Pooh," said Piglet. "I didn't plan it this way. It's just that some are thin and agile and some aren't."

"Rabbit's thin and agile, isn't he?" Pooh asked.

"Somehow I don't picture him Jumping and Squeaking," Pooh went on, hopefully. "Do you?"

"Now that you mention it, Pooh, I don't."

"Nor Kanga. Nor Owl or Eeyore."

"Especially not Eeyore," said Piglet.

Pooh cheered up. "Just as long as I'm not the only one. Well, now that we've learned our exercises, Piglet, let's go find Christopher Robin and have lunch, to protect ourselves from the hazard of Hollow Tummy."

"*Just* the thing," said Piglet.

5. EXERCISES THAT
GET SOMETHING DONE

Pooh refused to give up on the frisk. "Is there a Pudgy Frisk?" he asked me. "A Frisk of Little Brain? Or a Hummy Frisk?"

"Pooh, don't worry about Eeyore's exercises. Worry about yours."

"But I don't *have* any yet. I have a Shape, and I have a Hum about my Shape. But I don't have an exercise for it. Piglet can Jump and Squeak and Tigger bounces. What does a Pooh?"

Rabbit happened by, nodding smartly. "How are the exercises coming?" he asked.

"Slowly," I admitted. "Would you like to help out?"

"Perhaps. At a certain point. When I'm not too busy. What's that you're doing, Pooh?"

"The Pooh Frisk."

"Strange. You don't *look* frisky."

"It isn't working yet."

"Put your brain into it," Rabbit advised him. "More brain and less fluff! What are you doing now?"

Pooh was pulling on some thistles growing in a neat little patch. "I thought I'd bring these to Eeyore. In case he ran out of thistles today. You know how fond he is of thistles."

"Yes. Hallo, Piglet."

"Hallo, Rabbit," replied Piglet, ambling up.

"I must be off to Owl's," said Rabbit, and off he went.

"Rabbit doesn't seem much impressed with our workout," I observed.

"Look, Piglet," said Pooh. "I've been picking thistles for Eeyore."

"Is that your new exercise, Pooh?"

"No. It's just . . ." He turned to me, hopeful, bashful, and excited at once. "*Is* it my new exercise? I mean, could it be?"

"Picking thistles?"

"And I could help you, Pooh!" cried Piglet.

"Look—"

"It's very good for the tummy and the wrists," said Pooh, as he picked another thistle.

"And so simple," Piglet agreed. "You don't even need a diagram. You just find a basket—Pooh didn't, but next time he will—and then you set off."

"In a Hummy direction," Pooh added.

"Then you find a thistle patch . . ."

". . . and pick some!"

"Now, wait a minute—"

"And now for technique!" said Piglet, feeling rather proud of himself. "One bends at the knee or the waist, as one prefers."

Pooh bent, demonstrating.

"Thank you, Pooh. And use a graceful plucking motion with a good helping of elbow in it."

Pooh plucked.

"Now, Pooh, let's plan the box!"

Pooh visualized the title. " 'Gathering Thistles, an Exercise by Pooh and Piglet'!"

"Why *by* Pooh and Piglet?" I asked. "Why not *for?*"

"What do you mean?"

"Now that you've brought it up, **Gathering Thistles** is a perfectly decent exercise. It would work as well for the Piglet Shape as for the Pooh Shape, and it has the Attraction of Community Involvement, as you could present the thistles to Eeyore."

"I like the way the thistles sing when you hold them up to the breeze," Piglet noted.

"This is *much* Friendlier than frisking," said Pooh.

A NEW EXERCISE, COMPLETE WITH HUM

It got to be so friendly, that Pooh composed a Hum to Sustain One While Plucking:

> *"Guess where I'm going to, Piglet!"*
> *Says I.*
> *"Guess what I'm going to do!*
> *I'm gathering thistles for Eeyore to try.*
> *There's ever so many in view.*
> *Some taste like pepper,*
> *Some taste like steak,*
> *And some have the flavor of birthday cake.*
> *Where are you going to, Piglet?"*
> *Says he:*
> *"I'm gathering thistles with you!"*

We were so excited at the new-found sense of spontaneity in the workout that we rushed over to Eeyore to tell him about our new exercise and hand over the thistles.

"I'm sure you meant well," he said. "But these thistles are all bent."

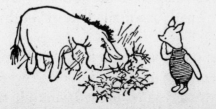

"I'm sorry, Eeyore," said Piglet. "But we didn't have a basket handy. Next time—"

"They don't taste right when they're bent," he said, sadly, pawing through them. "How would you like it if your food came all broken into little bits?"

The early reports on Gathering Thistles— Eeyore's report, at least—were so discouraging that Pooh and Piglet decided to cancel their box. But at least they were falling into an exercise frame-of-mind. I was congratulating myself especially on having won Piglet over when he asked me, "What good is exercise?"

I braced myself for another holdout action, and readied new arguments.

"I know it's supposed to keep me lively," he went on. "And it puts one's insides at their ease and makes one's outsides solid. But I can't help noticing that exercise does a lot more for the larger creatures than it does for me. They keep getting bigger and stronger—and bouncier—while I stay the same size."

"Well, you've only just started, Piglet. You have to give it a chance. Don't you at least feel better, all over? That's one immediate effect that exercise can have."

"Oh, I suppose so. I must say, it's very pleasant to walk home after an afternoon of Blowing Dandelions, knowing you've pushed yourself right to the limit. It makes one feel quite light-headed, almost like flying. But it doesn't seem to make me any taller. Or wider. Not that I want to be. But I have the feeling that it *should,* and it doesn't. And there it is."

"I must admit, the Piglet Shape, thin and agile as it is, does not put on weight easily."

"That's why I think there should be exercises that Accomplish Something on the Side, like our Thistle Gathering."

"For example?"

"Planting Haycorns."

"Ah."

"You see, digging a hole is good for your arm muscles, because of having to push the shovel in and out of the earth."

"So it is."

"And putting the haycorn into the hole has a kind of bending-over action in it, which presumably benefits the waist."

"Indeed."

"And then there's more shoveling, of course, to fill the hole again and cover the haycorn. And *then* you have to leap up and down on the dirt to flatten it."

"Let's see," I said. "Digging, bending over, more digging, and leaping up and down. That's an admirable workout, Piglet. There's something in it for every part of the body, all in one exercise."

"Best of all," he replied, "when the exercise is over, the haycorn grows up into an oak tree *filled* with haycorns. If you wait long enough."

"How long *do* you have to wait?"

Piglet looked doubtful. "I'm not sure. But I *think* Christopher Robin said it will take somewhat longer than a week from next April." He brightened. "Anyway, that leaves lots of time for planting more haycorns."

PLANTING HAYCORNS: TECHNIQUES AND TIPS

Grasping shovel firmly with both hands, dig wide, shallow hole. Hole should be handy to your haycorn storage area, but not immediately adjacent to anything in particular (to allow for growth of oak tree). Essential stylistic for this maneuver: *evenness of tempo.*

Carefully place haycorn in center of hole. Note shovel secured nearby in earth to avoid Training Accident. Essential stylistic for this maneuver: *concentration.*

Bound up and down upon the refilled hole. Be certain that the earth has been leveled off so other creatures will not lose their footing. The exercise is not over until there remains absolutely no sign that anything has been planted, to fool any passing Heffalumps (who regard planted haycorns as a delicacy). Essential stylistic for this maneuver: *pastoral abandon.*

"That's my idea of an Exercise," Piglet concluded. "Where you can Get Something Done while you go through your workout."

"What do you think, Pooh?" I asked.

"It would be nice to have something left over For Later," he agreed. "I often think that just after I've finished off a jar of hunny. But I don't know that I care all that much for an Accomplishment about a haycorn tree. Haycorns are very well in their way. They may be the best thing for those who like them. But not everybody does." He patted

Piglet's shoulder. "I just thought you ought to know."

"Oh, I quite agree," Piglet answered. "There's no accounting for some people's taste."

"Now, if we could work a different Accomplishment into an Exercise . . ."

"Such as what, Pooh?" I asked.

"There are many possibilities. But I was thinking . . . well, what about Filling Hunny Jars? Just for example, of course." He looked away. "It's one possibility." He scratched the ground with his paw. "Out of many."

"What would you fill the honey jars with, Pooh?" I asked.

He seemed surprised. "Why, hunny, of course!"

"Where would you get the honey to fill the jars with, Pooh?"

He was ready to withdraw the proposal on the spot. "Never mind," he said. "It was just a thought."

"Actually," I said, "there's something in that, Pooh. If you work it right, there's a good deal of exercise in filling a honey jar, and an Accomplishment as well—as the two of you gallantly proved on Eeyore's birthday one time."

Neither of them said anything, but Piglet's ears grew an arresting shade of pink and Pooh began to look off into the distance, as if he'd suddenly decided to wonder why a cow doesn't dance.

"I'm speaking," I went on, "about the celebrated **Balloon Bang Scramble**, one of the Forest's historic experiments in the field of physical culture and a truly interdisciplinary activity, taking in walking, running, lifting weights, and, best of all, improvisational dexterity!"

Pooh began to frown, as if he'd just realized that a cow possibly *might* dance when no one is looking, and then how could one be sure? Piglet's ears got pinker and pinker, and he glanced over at Pooh shyly, as if looking for a lesson in The Graceful Taking of Praise.

"What," asked Piglet, "was the Accomplishment?"

"A notable one: spreading birthday cheer. You remember, Piglet. Pooh had decided to give Eeyore a jar of honey for his birthday":

> It was a warm day, and he had a long way to go. He hadn't gone more than half-way when a sort of funny feeling began to creep all over him. It began at the tip of his nose and trickled all through him and out at the soles of his feet. It was just as if somebody inside him were saying, "Now then, Pooh, time for a little something."

"Dear, dear," said Pooh, "I didn't know it was as late as that." So he sat down and took the top off his jar of honey. "Luckily I brought this with me," he thought. "Many a bear going out on a warm day like this would never have thought of bringing a little something with him." And he began to eat.

"Now let me see," he thought, as he took his last lick of the inside of the jar, "where was I going? Ah, yes, Eeyore." He got up slowly.

And then, suddenly, he remembered. He had eaten Eeyore's birthday present!

"Bother!" said Pooh. "What *shall* I do? I *must* give him *something*."

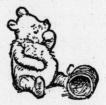

For a little while he couldn't think of anything. Then he thought: "Well, it's a very nice pot, even if there's no honey in it, and if I washed it clean, and got somebody to write *'A Happy Birthday'* on it, Eeyore could keep things in it, which might be Useful."

For his part, Piglet was just then heading toward Eeyore with a big red balloon:

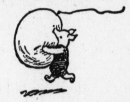

He held it very tightly against himself, so that it shouldn't blow away, and, running along, and thinking how pleased Eeyore would be, he didn't look where he was going . . . and suddenly he put his foot in a rabbit hole, and fell down flat on his face.

BANG!!!???***!!!

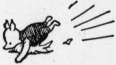

Piglet lay there, wondering what had happened. At first he thought that the whole world had blown up; and then he thought that perhaps only the Forest part of it had; and then he thought that perhaps only *he* had, and now he was alone in the moon or somewhere. And then he thought, "Well, even if I'm in the moon, I needn't be face downwards all the time," so he got cautiously up and looked about him.

He was still in the Forest!

"Well, that's funny," he thought. "I wonder what that bang was. I couldn't have made such a noise just falling down. And where's my balloon? And what's that small piece of damp rag doing?"

It was the balloon!

"Well," I noted, "what with Pooh's walk and Piglet's run, we've already logged a sound warmup. And then Pooh carried the honey jar, which is a form of what we call "power walking." It builds up the knuckles quite nicely, if you have knuckles. Do you, Pooh?"

"I'm not sure. I *think* I had some last week."

"What did we Accomplish in this exercise?" Piglet asked. "So far all we've done is empty a pot and ruin a balloon."

"And that's exactly where the Accomplishment comes in":

When Eeyore saw the pot, he became quite excited.

"Why!" he said. "I believe my Balloon will just go into that Pot!"

"Oh, no, Eeyore," said Pooh. "Balloons are much too big to go into Pots. What you do with a balloon is, you hold the balloon—"

"Not mine," said Eeyore proudly. "Look, Piglet!" And as Piglet looked sorrowfully round, Eeyore picked the balloon up with his teeth, and placed it carefully in the pot; picked it out and put it on the ground; and then picked it up again and put it carefully back.

"So it does!" said Pooh. "It goes in!"

"So it does!" said Piglet. "And it comes out!"

"Doesn't it?" said Eeyore. "It goes in and out like anything."

"I'm very glad," said Piglet happily, "that I thought of giving you Something to put in a Useful Pot."

But Eeyore wasn't listening. He was taking the balloon out, and putting it back again, as happy as could be . . .

"And the best thing of all," said Pooh, "is that this exercise contains a snack section right in the middle. Did you notice it? When I ate the hunny?"

Now, it's true that exercises as elaborate as the Scramble are unusual in any workout routine, partly because they seem to come off best only on birthdays and partly because even a well-appointed gym may not necessarily have balloons and honey jars on hand. And, saying that it did, still the Gym People might not be glad if you were to take these accoutrements out of their gym to go running around the countryside doing the Scramble.

There's also the worrisome question of how well the Scramble would work at times when no one you know is having a birthday. Christopher Robin brought this up, as being of strategic interest to the future of Forest fitness.

"Of course Pooh and Piglet and the others have rather more birthdays than people do elsewhere," he admitted. "But then suppose there had been a sudden rash of birthdays and they were all used up for that week?"

"That's right," said Pooh. "How would we do the Scramble?"

"We wouldn't," said Piglet.

"Ah," Pooh replied. "I thought there was an answer."

"What I want to know," asked Pooh, "is who gets the most out of the Balloon Bang Scramble?"

"I think Eeyore did," said Christopher Robin, "because he ended up with two birthday presents."

"That's true," Piglet agreed. "I can see that that's where the Accomplishment Section comes in. But I can't see putting a balloon into a jar and taking it out again as a useful exercise, no matter how often you do it. Certainly not as useful as Planting Haycorns."

"That depends on how you define useful," I said. "Remember, exercise isn't just a matter of Healthful Activity. It's also an approach to Feeling Good. And Eeyore certainly felt good about his birthday presents, didn't he?"

"Still," Piglet persisted, "he didn't run with a balloon, did he? In the exercise section?"

"Or walk," Pooh added, "with a heavy jar?"

"No . . ."

"Then," Piglet concluded, "who does get the most out of the Balloon Bang Scramble?"

"I expect the balloon does," said Pooh. And I expect he's right.

6. AN EXERCISE
FOR SAVAGE WEATHER

The Balloon Bang Scramble promised to be one of my most congenial suggestions—as Pooh put it, "Any exercise with a Hunny Section running right the way through it is an Exercise for Pooh."

"But what do we do in the winter, when it's too cold for picnics?" asked Piglet. "And when it's windy I can barely hear myself, much less the sky."

"When it's windy, you could take walks together as a kind of resistance exercise. Wind Walking. How does that sound, Piglet?"

"Like something I wouldn't be good at."

"Would it suit the Pooh Shape?" Pooh asked, still looking for an exercise he could make uniquely his.

"Absolutely, Pooh!"

Indeed, in **Wind Walking** the advantage lies in

two-legged height rather than in four-legged breadth. While wind walking, one uses one's weight to challenge and withstand the bluff breezes that blow in late autumn and early winter, when the trees have lost their foliage and the wind surges at will through glade and copse. At such times, even the Hundred Acre Wood, densely treed though it be, can become a center of howling, nipping blasts.

"Everyone can do it," said Pooh. "Though you ought to be a Bear of Great Strength before going out in the stronger winds."

"I wouldn't try it," Piglet agreed, "without Pooh being right there."

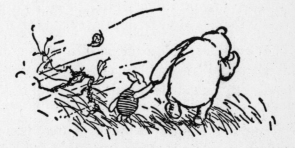

"And," Pooh went on, "you can do it anywhere. Anywhere there's wind, anyway. You just watch the way the tree branches are swaying to find the wind's direction, and then you march right into it."

I was thrilled to see Pooh taking a leading role in the dissemination of fitness in the Forest. "Any notes from the expert, Pooh?" I asked him. "To advise beginners?"

"Well, you have to keep your head lowered and hold your arms in. And keep moving. Also, take care of Piglet and have lots of fur."

"Good advice, that," said Piglet.

"Wind Walking is good for building up your strength," Pooh went on. "Beginners should start with a very small walk."

"Yes," Piglet agreed. "Like just around your house. Inside."

"No," I told him. "You have to start bigger than that. You could try it once a day from Pooh's to Kanga's and back again. Would that be right, Pooh?"

"It would, if you made sure to stop and visit with Kanga, Roo, and Tigger, to wish them a Friendly day and share a little smackerel of something."

"Right. And after a week of this, the walk would go more easily. Then you could try walking from your house to Kanga's and then on to Rabbit's. Wouldn't you say, Pooh?"

"Yes. And you could stop in at Rabbit's to ask him to demonstrate the different ways of opening tins of condensed milk." He blushed. "Just one, I mean."

"And later on, when great reserves of strength have been built up," I enthused, "you could try Wind Walking from Pooh's to Kanga's to Rabbit's and then all the way across the Forest to Christopher Robin's!"

"Yes!" Pooh chimed in, "and that would be the Friendliest wish of the day and the nicest smackerel of all!"

"I wonder," I said, "if you would want to swing down past the Hundred Acre Wood to Eeyore at Pooh Corner on your way back. I don't imagine you'd want to take a smackerel with Eeyore, though, as his idea of tea is boggy water and thistles and his idea of High Tea is more water and bigger thistles."

"Still," said Piglet, "what fun to wish him a Friendly day—though I must say the wind really blows through his part of the forest."

"Hallo, Eeyore," they called out cheerfully.

"Ah!" said Eeyore. "Lost your way?"

"We just came to see you," said Piglet. "And to see how your house was. Look, Pooh, it's still standing!"

"I know," said Eeyore. "Very odd. Somebody ought to have come down and pushed it over."

"We wondered whether the wind would blow it down," said Pooh.

"Ah, that's why nobody's bothered, I suppose. I thought perhaps they'd forgotten."

"Well, we're very glad to see you, Eeyore, and now we're going on to see Owl."

"That's right. You'll like Owl. He flew past a day or two ago and noticed me. He didn't actually say anything, mind you, but he knew it was me. Very friendly of him, I thought. Encouraging. Mind you don't get blown away, little Piglet. You'd be missed. People would say 'Where's little Piglet been blown to?'—really wanting to know. Well, good-bye. And thank you for happening to pass me."

EAR STREAMING

Variation techniques will help the walk go faster. Piglet, for example, has worked out an amusing method of streaming his ears in the air currents. This is, I confess, decorative rather than calisthenic. But sometimes one must allow oneself to be impelled by love of the sport as well as by practical needs.

Below, Piglet demonstrates the three major modes in **Ear Streaming**:

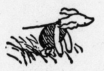

THE CARAVAN. Head kind of plonking on an angle, body moving quite slowly.
THINK OF: a sad little fish pensively swimming.

THE FLOUNCE. Head turning constantly to the sides, feet tracing irregular path.
THINK OF: a folk dance.

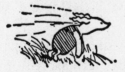

THE DART. Straight on and as fast as you can go.
THINK OF: lunch.

Pooh was so thrilled at discovering his own exercise that he developed another variation, Wind Walking Backwards, which amounts to Wind Walking While Looking Behind You.

"It makes a nice change," says Pooh, "from having the wind blowing in your face, though of course it's difficult to see where you are going."

"That's a problem, Pooh," I told him.

"Not if you're going nowhere in particular. Because then there wouldn't be much to see anyway, would there?"

WIND WALKING: HAZARDS AND GLORIES

"What about the hazards of Wind Walking?" I asked.

"Are there any?" answered Pooh.

"You could blow away, for one thing," Piglet offered. "As Eeyore says."

"Your hunny pots could blow away," Pooh added.

"Now that I think of it," said Piglet, "Wind Walking isn't as good for the Piglet Shape as I thought."

"Actually, Piglet, Wind Walking conditions on one occasion led to an extraordinary exercise that can *only* be done in the Piglet Shape. Remember, that very windy day at Owl's?"

"It was on just such a blustrous day as this," said Owl, "that my Uncle Robert, a portrait of whom you see upon the wall on your right, Piglet, while returning in the late forenoon from—What's that?"

There was a loud cracking noise.

"Look out!" cried Pooh. "Mind the clock! Out of

the way, Piglet! Piglet, I'm falling on you!"

"Help!" cried Piglet.

Pooh's side of the room was slowly tilting upwards and his chair began sliding down on Piglet's. The clock slithered gently along the mantelpiece, collecting vases along the way, until they all crashed together on to what had once been the floor, but was now trying to see what it looked like as a wall. Uncle Robert, who was going to be the new hearthrug, and was bringing the rest of the wall with him as carpet, met Piglet's chair just as Piglet was expecting to leave it, and for a little while it became very difficult to remember which was really the north. Then there was another loud crack ... Owl's room collected itself feverishly ... and there was silence.

In a corner of the room, the table-cloth began to wriggle.

Then it wrapped itself into a ball and rolled across the room. Then it jumped up and down once or twice, and put out two ears. It rolled across the room again, and unwound itself.

"Pooh," said Piglet nervously.

"Yes?" said one of the chairs.

"Did Owl *always* have a letter-box in his ceiling?"

I don't know about hunny pots or Piglet blowing away, but the wind certainly can break a big tree at its base and tumble a house over.

THE TABLECLOTH WRIGGLE

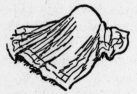

Off to a confident start.

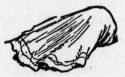

Proceeding smoothly.
(Note Rolling Haycorn
maneuver.)

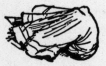

An unlucky spill.

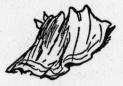

Recovery.

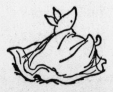

The athlete emerges triumphant.

"We can't go out by what used to be the front door," said Owl. "Something's fallen on it."

"But how else *can* you go out?" asked Piglet anxiously.

"That is the Problem, Piglet, to which I am asking Pooh to give his mind."

Pooh sat on the floor which had once been a wall, and gazed up at the ceiling which had once been another wall, with a front door in it which had once been a front door, and tried to give his mind to it.

"Could you fly up to the letter-box with Piglet on your back?" he asked.

"No," said Piglet quickly. "He couldn't."

"Because you see, Owl, if we could get Piglet into the letter-box, he might squeeze through the place where the letters come, and climb down the tree and run for help."

Piglet said hurriedly that he had been getting bigger lately, and couldn't *possibly,* much as he would like to, and Owl said he had had his letter-box made bigger lately in case he got bigger letters, so perhaps Piglet *might,* and suddenly an idea came to Pooh.

"Owl," said Pooh, "I have thought of something."

"Astute and Helpful Bear," said Owl.

Pooh looked proud at being called a stout and helpful bear, and said modestly that he just happened to think of it. You tied a piece of string to Piglet, and you flew up to the letter-box with the other end in your beak, and you pushed it through the wire and brought it down to the floor, and you and Pooh pulled hard at this end, and Piglet went slowly up the other end. And there you were.

"And there Piglet is," said Owl. "If the string doesn't break."

"Supposing it does?" asked Piglet, wanting to know.

"Then we try another piece of string."

This was not very comforting to Piglet, because however many pieces of string they tried pulling up with, it would always be the same him coming down.

"It won't break," whispered Pooh comfortingly, "because you're a Small Animal, and I'll stand underneath, and if you save us all, it will be a Very Grand Thing to talk about afterwards, and perhaps I'll make up a Song, and people will say 'It was so grand what Piglet did that a Respectful Pooh Song was made about it.' "

Piglet felt much better after this, and when he found himself slowly going up to the ceiling, he was so proud that he would have called out, "Look at *me!*" if he hadn't been afraid that Pooh and Owl would let go of their end of the string and look at him.

"Up we go!" said Pooh cheerfully.

"The ascent is proceeding as expected," said Owl helpfully. Piglet opened the letter-box and climbed in. Then, having untied himself, he began to squeeze into the slit, through which in the old days when front doors *were* front doors, many an unexpected letter that OWL had written to himself, had come slipping. He squeezed and he squoze, and then with one last squooze he was out.

"It's all right," he called through the letter-box. "Your tree is blown right over, Owl, and there's a branch across the door, but Christopher Robin and I can move it, and I'll go and tell him now. Goodbye, Pooh!"

A MAXIM FOR EXERCISE

"See, Piglet," I said. "It's not the Shape that matters in exercise—it's the spirit."

"Isn't there something *I* could do?" asked Pooh. "Something as Heroic as what Piglet did?"

"We'll find one, Pooh. You've got to keep at it. Pooh, you've got to *Go for the Hum!*"

He was transfixed. Confused, but transfixed. "The Hum?"

"The point is to extend yourself, Pooh, to broaden your physical experience—not just to feel how your body feels, but to Like How It Feels."

"The Hum?" he repeated.

"You know the way you feel when everything is going just right, and the trees are tall, and the sun is Friendly, and the wind is a whisper? And you don't feel pudgy?"

"Yes?"

"Going for the Hum makes the trees taller, the sun extra Friendly, and the wind like the whisper of a jar of honey, lonely in the cupboard."

"Go for the Hum," Pooh echoed.

"Can I Go for the Hum, too?" asked Piglet.

"Everyone can," I said. "But this isn't something you plan to do. The Hum creeps into the routine, *gradually* inspiring. Do you see what I mean?"

"Do you mean I'm still too pudgy?" asked Pooh.

"I mean it doesn't come easy until you work hard for it. The Hum is paradoxical. It's like a congratulation for things we have yet to accomplish."

"Go for the Hum," said Pooh.

"For the Hum," said Piglet.

"The Hum," said I.

Pooh nodded, took Piglet's hand, and started for home. "What Hum should we go for?" Piglet asked Pooh as they walked off.

" 'Cottleston Pie' might be a good place to start," said Pooh.

At last, I thought. At *last!* I'm finally getting through to them!

7. STRETCH-AND-FLEX EXERCISES

"I thought you would be coming over today," said Eeyore as Pooh and I walked up to him. "My neck muscles have been hurting all morning. I said to myself, 'It's either an approaching thunderstorm or approaching exercise.'"

"Now, Eeyore, Pooh has been looking for a special Poohish activity, and I've told him about the wonderful isometric purity of your **Donkey Balances**. I was hoping we could count on you for a practical demonstration."

"And I was hoping someone would come by with a candy cane tied up in a ribbon and say, 'Here, Eeyore, this is for you.' We can't all have our wish. Especially some of us."

"But I've been trying to Go for the Hum,"

Pooh explained. "And Donkey Balances sounded rather Hummy."

EXERCISE AS ACT OF WILL

The Donkey Balance is an ideal stretch-and-flex drill for the animal of middle weight, as it is not exhausting and can be repeated indefinitely, to the great profit of the leg muscles. The aim is to extend one hind leg up and forward to the ear, to push the ear flap upward very carefully with the extended leg, and to hold this position for twelve seconds. Rest, then repeat.

"You didn't tell them about the disadvantages," Eeyore put in.

"I didn't know there were any."

"That's right. Come crashing in without looking before you, and what happens?"

"What does happen?" asked Pooh.

"Just watch," Eeyore replied, and suddenly I realized what the main disadvantage of Donkey Balances is: they're so hard that even Eeyore can't do them.

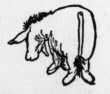
Step 1.
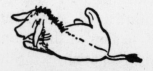
Step 2.

"It does aid the hearing," Eeyore told us as he got up and shook himself. "At least, it would if I could do them any time I wanted. Sometimes they work and sometimes they don't. Still, they're better than being buried in an avalanche."

"Are there other disadvantages, Eeyore?" I asked. "Now that we're on the subject?"

"Just one," he answered. "You can't do them on two legs."

"I can't?" cried Pooh.

"And you'd look silly, besides. Bears can't balance any more than Tiggers can fly."

Pooh turned to me. "Maybe I should wait a bit, till I'm a Bear of Great Strength."

"It takes four legs," Eeyore insisted, "and that's the whole of it. If you can't do it now, you can't do it later." He poked at a gorse twig that was spoiling the symmetry of a thistle patch. "No brains at all, some of them," he muttered.

"Come on, Pooh," I said. "Donkey Balances aren't the only stretch-and-flex exercise in the Forest."

"If you should see Christopher Robin, or Rabbit, or even Little Piglet," Eeyore called out as we were leaving, "you might tell him hello for me. None of them will care, but at least I tried. I met my Social Obligations."

I could tell by Pooh's particularly slow pace

that he had been crushed by this latest defeat. No matter what we tried, there seemed a distinct shortage of available exercises for the Pooh Shape. I feared that if I couldn't come up with something soon, he might give up altogether.

Sure enough, as we reached the Six Pine Trees he said, "It's no good—*that's* what it is. Or isn't. I just can't find my special exercise."

"Now, Pooh. You've got to be patient."

"But I *have* been."

"Pooh, you've just begun!"

"Everyone has an exercise but me."

"Pooh—"

"Even Eeyore has exercises. Piglet doesn't like exercises and *he* has some he can do. But I don't." Suddenly a fir-cone flew down at our feet, and Christopher Robin came running up.

"*I* threw it, Bear," he said, hugging Pooh. "Shall we have a game?"

"All right," said Pooh.

"What's the matter?" Christopher Robin asked Pooh. Then he looked at me. "Aren't the exercises getting on well, then?"

"Well . . . not entirely," I admitted.

"I'm not surprised to hear it," said Rabbit, who had suddenly and perhaps even stealthily joined us. "It's not being Organized properly. Anyone can see that."

Christopher Robin and Pooh were gathering an artillery of fir-cones.

"It wants categories," Rabbit went on. "Point systems. Championships. Winners and losers. It's no good just putting a foot in the water. You've got to swim or sink."

Piglet came up, traded hallos, and immediately began to join Christopher Robin and Pooh in their game of throwing fir-cones about.

"Without Organization you don't have anything," Rabbit persisted.

Watching the others tossing their cones, I sensed that the solution to Pooh's problem was at hand.

"Exercise is like anything else," Rabbit concluded. "It has a beginning, a middle, and an end. And it's best to proceed in that order."

"Pooh!" I cried. "Why didn't I think of this before? You've already got a perfectly acceptable stretch-and-flex right here! Pooh: *you have an exercise!*"

EXERCISE AS GAME

Obviously, **Throwing Fir-cones** consists in . . . well, throwing fir-cones. But how many? How often? In which direction? How far? Is there a target, or is it a freestyle toss without purpose?

All this is left to the sportsman's choice. Some use Throwing Fir-cones as a filler exercise, between heavier activities. Others build an entire workout around it.

"I like the choosing of the cones," Pooh tells me. "It's like a warmup time, collecting a great pile of them."

"I only gather a few cones," says Piglet. "They're all pretty much the same."

"They are exactly the same," says Rabbit. "Just pick up the first five cones you see, and there's an end to Bother."

"I like to help Pooh," says Christopher Robin, "because he's so serious about it."

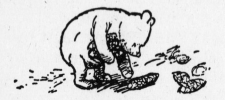

The four of them then hold a friendly contest to see who can throw the farthest, or the highest, or in the most squiggly patterns. Usually everybody wins. It's that sort of contest.

Tigger and Roo have their own version, which they call **Coners**. This has no warmup. Instead of collecting specific fir-cones, they walk around until they find a whole lot of them waiting.

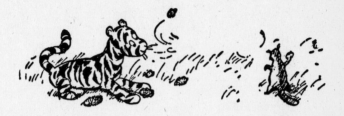

Then Tigger stands off about three feet from Roo, and Roo throws cones at Tigger, and Tigger throws cones back at Roo. Kanga often comes along, mainly to say things like, "Now, Roo dear, just one more throw and we ought to be getting back for your medicine."

OWL AND EXERCISE

Owl had been keeping himself Separate from Exercise, though on occasion I would surprise him In Consultation with Rabbit. I thought Throwing Fir-cones might give Owl the most practical entree into exercise, and invited him to join us.

"No, thank you," he proclaimed. "I must consider vetting my party list."

"Well," I went on encouragingly, "anytime you want to try throwing a fir-cone—"

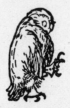

Figure A.
A highlight of Owl's Daily Constitutional:
One foot's up and one foot's down.

"Those who can spell Thursday do not throw fir-cones! Besides, I have already instituted the appropriate Daily Constitutional." (See Figure A.)

"Ah. Yes. Well . . . all right, Owl. Carry on."

The main thing was, Pooh had an exercise. Not a real exercise, not the special Pooh Exercise for Becoming a Bear of Great Strength. But this would do until something better came along.

8. WATER SPORTS

The Forest boasts many natural watercourses, of various sizes and personalities. There are the spirited brooklets that dart impatiently along as if they can't wait to see what it's like when they get to wherever it is they're going. There is the imperturbable stream that meanders through Eeyore's bog in a highly messy manner, as if no one had ever settled the question of which was supposed to be the wet part and which the dry—not to the stream's satisfaction. Then there is the impressive river that runs down the very center of the Forest, racing over rocks, swirling into pools, growing grander and slower as it passes through the Hundred Acre Wood, and at last widening to move with tactful majesty under the big wooden bridge at the

Forest's edge, where Pooh devised the game called
Poohsticks.

GAME AS EXERCISE?

I toyed with the idea of encouraging Pooh by letting him claim Poohsticks as his special exercise.
After all, not only did Pooh invent it, but it would
be unthinkable in the Forest to play it without him.
Pooh *is* Poohsticks, his spirit the very spirit of the
game. Even when he doesn't win, he remains the
game's essential player.

In the end, however, I decided against letting
Pooh build his Daily Routine around Poohsticks. If
I were to bring him around, it would have to be in
strictly athletic terms.

Still, there is a place for Poohsticks in one's
workout, provided one uses it as a kind of post-
calisthenic warmdown, or an All Together Now finale, to see the day to its close.

THE PLAYING OF POOHSTICKS

Poohsticks provides an admirably social exercise: any number may play. Pooh even played it by
himself on the day of its invention, and he started
with fir-cones instead of sticks. One must have a
bridge, however.

"That's funny," said Pooh. "I dropped the cone on the other side and it came out on this side! I wonder if it would do it again?" And he went back for some more fir-cones.

It did. It kept on doing it. Then he dropped two in at once, and leant over the bridge to see which of them would come out first; and one of them did; but as they were both the same size, he didn't know if it was the one which he wanted to win, or the other one. So the next time he dropped one big one and one little one, and the big one came out first, which was what he had said it would do, and the little one came out last, which was what he had said it would do, so he had won twice . . . and when he went home for tea, he had won thirty-six and lost twenty-eight, which meant that he was—that he had—well, you take twenty-eight from thirty-six, and *that's* what he was. Instead of the other way round.

And that was the beginning of the game called Poohsticks, which Pooh invented, and which he and his friends play on the edge of the Forest.

"I still don't see why I can't call Poohsticks my exercise," Pooh grumbled as I was quizzing him on data and technique. "It's my game, isn't it?"

"That's the problem, Pooh. It *is* a game. It's not an exercise. But don't worry: Poohsticks holds a prominent page in the catalogue of Forest Sport. Speaking of which, how about some expert advice for the novice?"

"In a box?"

And here it is:

POOH'S TIPS FOR BEGINNERS

1. Sticks work better than cones because you can tell them apart, while fir-cones tend to resemble each other quite fiercely.
2. Try to choose a Hummy sort of stick—the kind that seems to be looking for a Rhyme.

IMMERSION: PASTIME OR DUTY?

Poohsticks would probably be of greater athletic value if the animals themselves took part in the race instead of leaving the contest to their sticks. But then **Swimming** is not a Forest specialty. It's something most of our friends save for an unusual occasion, such as unintentionally falling into a river.

Only Roo actively indulges in swimming, and even he went in for the first time quite by accident, on the celebrated all-Forest Expotition to Discover the North Pole:

Roo was washing his face and paws in the stream, while Kanga explained to everybody proudly that this was the first time he had ever washed his face himself.

"I don't hold with all this washing," grumbled Eeyore. "This modern Behind-the-ears nonsense. What do *you* think, Pooh?"

"Well," said Pooh, "*I* think—"

But we shall never know what Pooh thought, for there came a sudden squeak from Roo, a splash, and a loud cry of alarm from Kanga.

"So much for *washing*," said Eeyore.

"Roo's fallen in!" cried Rabbit, and he and Christopher Robin came rushing down to the rescue.

"Look at me swimming!" squeaked Roo from the middle of his pool, and was hurried down a waterfall into the next pool.

"Are you all right, Roo dear?" called Kanga anxiously.

"Yes!" said Roo. "Look at me sw—" and down he went over the next waterfall into another pool.

Everybody was doing something to help. Piglet was jumping up and down making "Oo, I say" noises; Owl was explaining that the Important Thing was to keep the Head Above Water; Kanga was jumping along the bank, saying "Are you *sure* you're all right, Roo dear?" to which Roo, from whatever pool he was in at the moment, was answering "Look at me swimming!"

"All right, Roo, I'm coming," called Christopher Robin.

"Get something across the stream lower down, some of you fellows," called Rabbit.

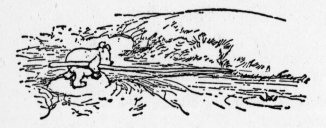

But Pooh was getting something. Two pools below Roo he was standing with a long pole in his paws, and Kanga came up and took one end of it, and between them they held it across the lower part of the pool; and Roo, still bubbling proudly, "Look at me swimming," drifted up against it, and climbed out.

"Did you see me swimming?" squeaked Roo excitedly, while Kanga scolded him and rubbed him down. "Pooh, did you see me swimming? That's called swimming, what I was doing. Rabbit, did you see what I was doing? Swimming. Christopher Robin, did you see me—"

But Christopher Robin wasn't listening. He was looking at Pooh.

"Pooh," he said, "where did you find that pole?"

Pooh looked at the pole in his hands.

"I just found it," he said. "I just picked it up."

"Pooh," said Christopher Robin solemnly, "the Expedition is over. You have found the North Pole!"

"Oh!" said Pooh.

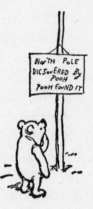

Roo is so enthusiastic about swimming that when he happens near a stream he might need to fall in accidentally, because Kanga isn't quite as enthusiastic about streams as Roo is. "I must say," she told me, "I think Roo gets all the exercise he needs by jumping in and out of mouse holes in his sandy-pit playgrounds." (This is not to mention leaping from chair to chair at the picnic table, and having hiccoughs, two of Roo's most constant activities.)

But Roo has become the Forest's unrivaled champion at one exercise, **Avoiding a Bath.**

This is a favorite exercise in the Forest, but Roo gets more practice than anyone because of his proximity to Kanga. "Now Roo, dear," Kanga will say, "it's time for your bath"—and so the workout begins, as Roo thinks of excuses and postponements and Kanga deftly rebuts them.

It may seem odd that Roo likes to get into water in the natural environment and objects to it when it's located all in one place (such as the bathtub). But then what feels like sport in one setting can feel like Bother in another.

Avoiding a bath is a saturation exercise, like pushups: you can't do too much of it. Experts agree it is wise to keep moving at all times and to verbalize every pretext that comes to mind, no matter how feeble. "I'm allergic to water!" Roo will squeal, or "Shouldn't I be visiting Alexander Beetle just now?" or even "Help!" The fact that Roo has invariably ended up in the bath thus far should not discourage newcomers from this exercise, for it strengthens the will even as it tests mind and muscles.

However, one should work up to the feat, not start out cold. Piglet once found himself in Roo's place at bath-time, and made the two mistakes of standing still *and* attempting to reason his way out of the water:

"Kanga, I see the time has come to speak plainly," said Piglet.

"Funny little Roo," said Kanga, as she got the bath-water ready.

"I am *not* Roo," said Piglet loudly. "I am Piglet!"

"Yes, dear, yes," said Kanga soothingly. "And imitating Piglet's voice, too! So clever of him," she went on, as she took a large bar of yellow soap out of the cupboard. "What *will* he be doing next?"

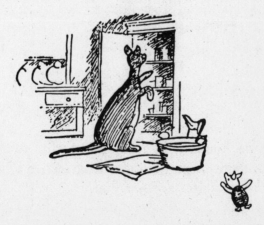

"Can't you *see?*" shouted Piglet. "Haven't you got *eyes?* Look at me!"

"I *am* looking, Roo, dear," said Kanga rather severely. "And you know what I told you yesterday about making faces. If you go on making faces like Piglet's, you will grow up to *look* like Piglet—and *then* think how sorry you will be. Now then, into the bath, and don't let me have to speak to you about it again."

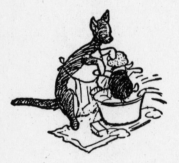

Thus we see the folly of getting into a fitness cycle without adequate preparation. In avoiding a bath, footwork and patter are essential.

EEYORE-IN-WATER

    I wondered if Eeyore ever goes in for a swim.

    "Swimming?" he said. "Bubbles in the nose,

soggy hide, tail all shrunken and wrinkled, that sort of thing?"

"Well . . ."

"Foolishness. Waste. Nothing in it, if you ask me. Not that anybody ever does."

"*I'm* asking you, Eeyore."

"I don't like it."

"Yet it was you who introduced **The Pooh-sticks Float.**"

He sniffed. "For all the good it did me."

"I must say, Eeyore, you do it awfully well. Though it surely was a shock that first time, when you came sailing out under the bridge instead of the Poohsticks":

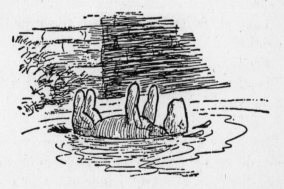

"Eeyore, what *are* you doing there?" said Rabbit.

"I'll give you three guesses, Rabbit. Digging holes in the ground? Wrong. Leaping from branch to branch of a young oak-tree? Wrong. Waiting for somebody to help me out of the river? Right. Give Rabbit time, and he'll always get the answer."

"But, Eeyore," said Pooh in distress, "what can we—I mean, how shall we—do you think if we—"

"Yes," said Eeyore. "One of those would be just the thing. Thank you, Pooh."

"I grant you, the Float is a relatively esoteric exercise in that one is first involuntarily bounced into the water by Tigger, then drifts helplessly along on one's back till rescued. Still, it's a pleasant way to loosen up in the water."

"Bad for the ears," Eeyore noted.

"Oh?"

"They get waterlogged. Then the flaps don't work right."

"The flaps?"

"On the ears. To hear with? If there's anything worth hearing?"

"Oh."

"No doubt it seems like some modern wonder-cure to you, eddying about with one's legs in the air like a bathing toy. But it did not do any wonders for me. Not," he concluded, "that I noticed."

"Still, you did enliven the Poohsticks contest that day."

"Anything to oblige," he snorted. "Next time

you're short a doormat, be sure to send for me."

"I'd rather send for you to pass on the secrets of your technique to those who are trying the Float for the first time. You might offer a master class in Freshwater Recreation."

"Well ... of course, there's a secret to everything—if you do it *well*, I mean."

"How about sharing yours?"

"It's nothing, really. Just a sort of ... sort of a ... floating motion ..."

"I suppose the mechanics of the thing are what really make it go."

"Instinct has something to do with it, too," he admitted, pacing among his thistles in what was for him a rather stately manner. "A sensitivity about Why We're Here and How to Feel When We Go Somewhere Else."

"Any procedural points we should know about?"

"Keep your back straight. That's the thing."

"Straight back."

"The legs should be aimed directly upward."

"Legs up."

"And no larking about. It's a float, not a water ballet. It isn't supposed to be fun; it's supposed to be good for you."

"But didn't you enjoy it at all?"

"I believe I would rate it somewhere between

eating a bar of carbolic soap and sitting on a porcu-
pine. But we didn't have a tornado that day. Let's
always try to look on the bright side of the matter."

POOH–IN–WATER I: THE BEE CHASE

"Do you ever swim, Pooh?" I asked him.

"Sometimes. By chance. And not in water unless I can't help it."

"When can't you help it?"

"During The Bee Chase."

"The Bee Chase? Already titled and everything?"

"Well, that's what I call it. The bees may call
it something else."

The Bee Chase, it turns out, is an interdisciplinary athletic designed to merge the pleasures of
running with those of aquatics.

"It's not designed," Pooh puts in. "It just happened."

I beg Pooh's pardon. The Bee Chase begins
quietly, even stealthily, as the athlete approaches
the honey hives in the Hundred Acre Wood.

"Be sure to supply yourself with an empty
hunny pot," Pooh warns. "You never know when
one might come in handy."

"Pooh, why don't you tell us about The Bee

Chase yourself? After all, it's you teaching me on this one, not the other way around."

"Well, you sort of follow your nose. Then there's a little mucking about in the bush and climbing a tree or so . . . Isn't this a good exercise?"

"So far."

"It gets better. Anyway, after the mucking and climbing—so you can get to know the Forest better—you come to the hunny hives. And of course where there's hunny hives there's usually hunny. The next thing after that, unfortunately, is the bee part.

"Now comes the running section of the exercise, as you head for the stream that runs through the wood. The bees usually run along with you."

"Pooh, what pace would you recommend here? Jogging? Trotting? A crisp canter?"

"I go as fast as I can."

"Right. Wind sprints. I gather, then, that admiring the natural beauty of the scene bathed in happy weather is less important than reaching water as soon as possible?"

"Yes. Run for the water."

"And when the athlete reaches the water?"

"He should jump in."

"Effecting thereby a Sudden Temporary Immersion of the Body."

"What?"

"Never mind, Pooh. What's next?"

"Well, when he's under water, he should stroke downstream a bit before coming up for air. This makes it less interesting for the bees, and they usually fly back to their hive."

"Well, Pooh," I commented, "it would seem that The Bee Chase is very good for the legs, what with all the mucking, climbing, running, and swimming. And I notice that it includes its own cooling-off maneuver at the end. I don't think we've found the key Pooh exercise yet, but we're coming along nicely."

"I wonder if The Bee Chase is good for a Daily Routine, though."

"Oh?"

"Well, if you tried it every day, the bees would be certain to catch on sooner or later. They would Notice Something."

"How smart of you, Pooh, to point that out."

"They could take to waiting by the stream for you to come up for air. They could buzz angrily at you. They might even sting. You never know with bees."

"Keen thinking, Pooh."

"Supposing it's a special exercise, too?" says Pooh. "Not a run-and-swim for just any day, but a run-and-swim for a . . . well, a day that . . . a kind of . . ."

"A kind of run-and-swim day?"

"Yes," he agrees. "I'd forgotten the exact term for it."

It's the kind of day, I would guess, with a taste of snapdragon in the air, when the Hums of Pooh begin to run through your head. A Hummy Sort of Day.

But Pooh, my increasingly indispensable advisor on matters pertaining to Forest culture, asks, "What if it's *not* a Hummy Sort of Day?"

"Why don't you make up a box about it?"

THREE THINGS TO DO INSTEAD OF THE BEE CHASE IF IT'S NOT A HUMMY SORT OF DAY

1. Track the Spotted or Herbaceous Backson.
2. Explore the Hundred Acre Wood (but don't get lost).
3. Ask Owl to spell "Cottleston Pie."

POOH–IN–WATER II: THE FLOATING BEAR

The novelty of water sports wears off somewhat once you realize that it's all either swimming or floating. However, the always resourceful Pooh developed a variation he calls **The Hunny Pot Paddle**. Some exercises are for health, some for fun, some for a Very Important Mission. The Hunny Pot Paddle is the Mission kind.

It's quite famous, perhaps even historical, for Pooh devised it In Time of Flood:

> He took his largest pot of honey and escaped with it to a broad branch of his tree, well above the water, and then he climbed down again and escaped with another pot . . . and when the whole Escape was finished, there was Pooh sitting on his branch, dangling his legs, and there beside him, were ten pots of honey . . .

Four days later, there was Pooh with ten empty honey pots, when a bottle floated by. There was a message in it which Pooh couldn't quite make out, not being able to read. Anyway, the main thing was not what the message said but that the bottle *floated:*

> "If a bottle can float, then a jar can float, and if a jar floats, I can sit on the top of it, if it's a very big jar."

> So he took his biggest jar, and corked it up. "All boats have to have a name," he said, "so I shall call mine *The Floating Bear.*" And with these words he dropped his boat into the water and jumped in after it.

For a little while Pooh and The Floating Bear were uncertain as to which of them was meant to be on the top, but after trying one or two different positions, they settled down with The Floating Bear underneath and Pooh triumphantly astride it, paddling vigorously with his feet.

"To get Christopher Robin," Piglet chimed in, "and then to rescue me! Because I sent the message in the bottle."

"The handy thing about the Hunny Pot Paddle," Pooh noted, "is that you don't have to have a flood to do it."

"Of course."

"But it helps. And of course, it also helps to be a Bear of Great Strength."

"*Pooh!* You've found your Special Exercise!"

"I *have?*"

"The Hunny Pot Paddle! There you are, Pooh—you invented it, you made history with it, and only you can do it!"

Pooh looked down so as not to look overbearing (if you see what I mean), but it was His Moment, and, clearly, he knew it. "Only *I* could do it?" he finally asked.

"Only you."

"I, Pooh Bear?"

"Absolutely."

THE HUNNY POT PADDLE
IN THREE EASY STEPS

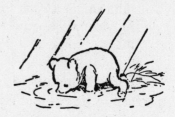

Step 1.

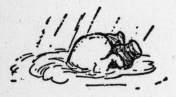

Step 2.

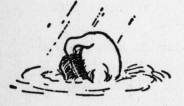

Step 2a.

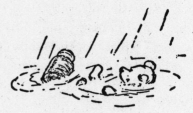

Step 2b.

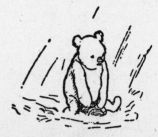

Step 2c.

Step 3.

"Does that mean I'm not pudgy anymore?"

"It means that you are and always have been The Dauntless Floating Bear of the Pleasurable Pooh Shape, Esquire."

Trying to appear decently modest, Pooh said, "I could try to teach the others about The Hunny Pot Paddle. They possibly wouldn't be good at it, of course, but I could *try* to teach them. So as not to be selfish."

"Tremendous, Pooh! Now, what size pot do you recommend?"

"Oh, hunny size or so."

"I would prefer to do it on a smaller pot," said Piglet. "Like the kind flowers come in. Though I'd really prefer not to do it at all."

"Well, Piglet, what water sports do you prefer, then?"

"Watching the others swim," he replied.

9. MAKING UP PERSONAL
WORKOUT CHARTS

"Here," said Piglet, handing me a sheet of paper. "I thought you would like this."

"What is it?"

"It's a list. Like what Rabbit makes up when he Organizes."

"A list of what?"

"Oh, you'll see. I have to go now. I promised Rabbit I'd meet him at Owl's."

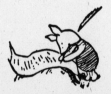

Piglet's list was a surprise:

PIGLET'S WORKOUT, BY PIGLET (ME)

WARMUP: Think about exercise.

FIRST EXERCISE: Be tidy. Plan ahead. Choose the second exercise.

SECOND EXERCISE: Concentrate. Repeat first exercise.

THIRD EXERCISE: Take a short nap, to avoid exhaustion.

FOURTH EXERCISE: Check Piglet Shape in mirror. Are all your calories in place?

FIFTH EXERCISE: Don't get discouraged.

SIXTH EXERCISE: Optional.

I was touched. An actual Daily Exercise Routine. Granted, it was on the loose side—but attitude matters more than anything in the first stage, after all.

Scarcely had I absorbed Piglet's surprise than Christopher Robin ambled up and handed me another list.

"Exercises?" I asked.

"How did you know?"

"Just a hunch."

"I'll see you later. I have to meet Rabbit at Owl's."

"Tell me something. Whose idea was it to make up these lists?"

"Oh, I just thought you'd like it."

MY EXERCISES
FIRST EXERCISE: Imitating a train.
SECOND EXERCISE: Going to India.
THIRD EXERCISE: Coming home (by lunchtime).
FOURTH EXERCISE: Walking nowhere with Pooh.
REST PERIOD: Telling Pooh about India.
FIFTH EXERCISE: Walking back.

Even more surprising than a list from Piglet or Christopher Robin was one for Roo and Tigger, obviously made with Kanga's assistance. She bounded by as I was taking the shade in the Hundred Acre Wood, Roo in her pocket and Tigger crashing along, now ahead, now behind.

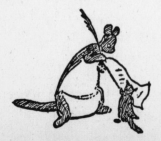

"Roo and Tigger thought you might be glad to read this," she said, handing it to me.

"It's about me, you know," Roo proudly squeaked. "And Tigger!"

"We told what to say," Tigger told me.

"You mean, 'We *dictated* it,' Tigger," said Kanga in a correcting tone.

"You didn't," Tigger replied. "*We* did."

"Thank you," I said. "I guess this is my day for lists."

Kanga smiled knowingly and hopped away with her young. Their list had a certain purity:

Coners the splunk and swimming then bouncing and getting bounced also running, and you can do some of these twice.

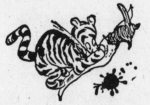

At last there remained Pooh, virtually my protégé as the Bear of Great Strength, more or less intrepidly assembling his Daily Routine as he Goes for the Hum. When I saw him stumping up with a piece of paper in his paw I had to suppress a grin of triumph.

"Something for me, Pooh?"

"Yes. It's a surprise."

"Everything is, today."

He stood by as I began to study it. "Couldn't you read it aloud?"

So I did:

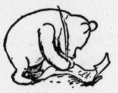

POOH'S ACTIVITIES

WARMUP: Counting pots of hunny.

THEN: Having some.

FIRST EXERCISE: Save some for later.

HOW MUCH?: A little.

SECOND EXERCISE: Have the rest. (This is later, now.)

THIRD EXERCISE: The Hunny Pot Paddle. (Sing ho! for Pooh!)

UNLESS: It isn't wet out.

Christopher Robin helped Pooh.

"Well?" he asked. "Do you like it?"

"I . . . love the thought. But, Pooh, do counting honey pots and eating honey *really* belong in an exercise program?"

"I always do them, though. Isn't exercise something you always do?"

"Not something you'd always do anyway. Exercise is something you go out of your way to do because . . . well, because . . ."

"Because you have to?"

"Because you *want* to."

"I was afraid it would be something like that," he said sadly. "Because what if I would rather not?"

"Then I don't know. Maybe then you shouldn't exercise."

He seemed completely baffled.

"Go on to Owl's now," I told him. "I'll meet you there."

I went to Eeyore's first. I might as well pick up the workout lists, if the Forest was going to make them up. However, Eeyore had no list, and I can't say he felt very progressive about the subject.

"A balanced diet of thistles and grass and the odd frisk here and there is all they need," he announced. I sensed the implication that "they" didn't know what was good for them. "What the Forest wants," he added, "is brains, not muscles. Thinking first—*then* comes playtime."

"*There* you are," said Rabbit, walking up.

"Splendid. I've been looking for you."

"I see you have a list, too."

"Yes. For our new group. The Forest Exercise Club. At Owl's. We're Organizing and Planning. Here." He handed me his list. "Oh, hallo, Eeyore. You're here, too."

"Yes, Rabbit. I'm here, too. No doubt it *is* surprising of me to turn up in my own habitat. No wonder it took you so long to notice me. It's foolish and stubborn of me to live somewhere, perhaps, but we all have our little caprices, don't we?"

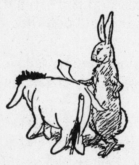

"I must get on," said Rabbit. "They'll be waiting for me." And away he went.

"What are they up to?" I wondered aloud.

"Perhaps someone's giving a party," said Eeyore.

"We would surely have been invited, if that were the case."

"One of us, at any rate. Some others might not have been." He sniffed at a lone thistle poking out from the base of a birch tree. "But I don't mind. Not being invited to a party saves one from not having a good time at a party. If it's not one thing, it's another."

As he nibbled his thistle, I examined Rabbit's list:

PROGRAM ON PLANNING EXERCISES

1. *Introductory statement.* There is Exercise in the Forest.
2. *However.* Some like it and some don't.
3. *Not to mention.* Some are good at it and some are not.
4. Such as Tigger. (Good at it, also likes it.)
5. *A question.* Does the Forest need Exercise?
6. Questioning by Rabbit on this and related topics has revealed a variety of answers. (See 3.)
7. Also see 2.
8. With the lingering impression that:
9. *There is not as much enthusiasm about exercise as Some People think.*

No sooner had I digested this than Rabbit came back. "Forgot to tell you," he said. "The Forest Exercise Club are planning a competition or so. It's going to be quite famous. Everybody will be talking about it, even the beetles. You might drop by Owl's if you're in the mood."

"Rabbit, just what is going on here?"

"I'll see you at Owl's," he said, quite satisfied that he was Busy and Important.

"Pardon me," said Eeyore, as I watched Rabbit vanish into the Forest. "Do you have to stand right on top of the nicest thistle patch about?"

"Eeyore, I'm going to Owl's."

"That's right. The party. Be sure to tell them all thank you for saving me the inconvenience of not enjoying myself."

"Eeyore, it's not a party, believe me. It's an exercise club, and I'm sure you're welcome any time."

"That's all very well, but you've ruined my thistle patch."

10. THE FOREST
EXERCISE CLUB

When I got to Owl's, I found Owl, Rabbit, and Piglet watching Pooh helping Christopher Robin get in and out of his boots.

"What's all this?" I asked.

"It's a new exercise," Christopher Robin told me. "Rabbit taught us."

"Anyone can do it," Piglet enthused. "Regardless of Shape, if you know what I mean."

"Rabbit taught you?" I turned to him. "Since when have you taken an interest in exercise?"

"Rabbit has generously lent his Inventive Genius to the formation of the Forest Exercise Club," Owl explained. "Owl, Most Honorary President and Secretary. Rabbit, Author of Exercises. And, if you'll excuse me," he added, "I must get back to my Exercise Diagrams."

"All right, show me your new exercise," I said, as Owl went inside.

"Pooh, a Demonstration," said Rabbit. "Piglet, you stand aside like a good fellow. And now: **Putting on Big Boots**. Two are needed," Rabbit explained, as Pooh and Christopher Robin demonstrated. "One, naturally, puts them on. And the other—"

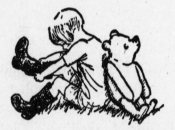

"The other doesn't," observed Pooh.

"What the other does," Rabbit continued, "the other being Pooh, as you can see, is to lean. At the same time, Christopher Robin pushes against Pooh. Meanwhile *putting on the boots!*"

"And what's that supposed to be?"

"That's Putting on Big Boots," Christopher Robin replied, "by the Forest Exercise Club."

"If you insist. But what about the data? Don't we get something about Leverage? Weight Balance? Sets and Reps? Timing?" I was hoping to show them that they couldn't get on without me as easily as Rabbit seemed to think.

"I gave you all the facts," said Rabbit. "One puts on the boots, and the other doesn't."

"Well, I'm glad to see you all coming up with exercises without my help. Now, as long as we're all here together, why don't we start with some frisk warmups and then—"

"This is the Forest Exercise Club," said Rabbit. "We only do special Forest Exercises here."

"Frisking is a Forest exercise. Eeyore developed it."

"*You* developed it, actually. Eeyore just does it."

"Why don't we tell about the **Woozle Walk**?" asked Christopher Robin. "Pooh and Piglet were the first to do it," Christopher Robin explained. "But I discovered it. Because I watched them."

One fine winter's day when Piglet was brushing away the snow in front of his house, he happened to look up, and there was Winnie-the-Pooh. Pooh was walking round and round in a circle, thinking of something else, and when Piglet called to him, he just went on walking.

"Hallo!" said Piglet, "what are *you* doing?"

"Hunting," said Pooh.

"Hunting what?"

"Tracking something," said Winnie-the-Pooh very mysteriously.

"Tracking what?" said Piglet, coming closer.

"I shall have to wait until I catch up with it," said Winnie-the-Pooh. "Now, look there." He pointed to the ground in front of him. "What do you see there?"

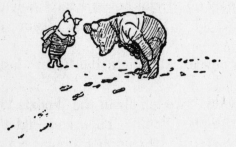

"Tracks," said Piglet. "Paw-marks." He gave a little squeak of excitement. "Oh, Pooh! Do you think it's a—a—a Woozle?"

"Notice that the Woozle Walk cannot be done alone," said Rabbit.

"At least not by a Very Small Animal of the Piglet Shape," Piglet agreed.

Pooh went on tracking, and Piglet, after watching

him for a minute or two, ran after him. Winnie-the-Pooh had come to a sudden stop, and was bending over the tracks in a puzzled sort of way.

"What's the matter?" asked Piglet.

"It's a very funny thing," said Bear, "but there seem to be *two* animals now. This—whatever-it-was—has been joined by another—whatever-it-is—and the two of them are now proceeding in company. Would you mind coming with me, Piglet, in case they turn out to be Hostile Animals?"

There was a small spinney of larch trees just here, and it seemed as if the two Woozles, if that is what they were, had been going round this spinney; so round this spinney went Pooh and Piglet after them; Piglet passing the time by telling Pooh what his Grandfather Trespassers W had done to Remove Stiffness after Tracking, and how his Grandfather Trespassers W had suffered in his later years from Shortness of Breath, and other matters of interest, and Pooh wondering what a Grandfather was like, and if perhaps this was Two Grandfathers they were after now, and, if so, whether he would be allowed to take one home and keep it, and what Christopher Robin would say. And still the tracks went on in front of them . . .

Suddenly Winnie-the-Pooh stopped, and pointed excitedly in front of him. *"Look!"*

"What?" said Piglet, with a jump. And then, to

show that he hadn't been frightened, he jumped up and down once or twice in an exercising sort of way.

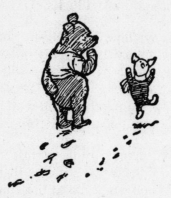

"The tracks!" said Pooh. *"A third animal has joined the other two!"*

"Pooh!" cried Piglet. "Do you think it is another Woozle?"

"No," said Pooh, "because it makes different marks. It is either Two Woozles and one, as it might be, Wizzle, or Two, as it might be, Wizzles and one, if so it is, Woozle. Let us continue to follow them."

"Walking around a few trees?" I said. "This is what the Forest Exercise Club calls exercise?"

"But this is no ordinary walk," said Pooh. "It's a Surprising Hike."

"A Great Event," Rabbit added.

All of a sudden, Winnie-the-Pooh stopped again, and licked the tip of his nose in a cooling manner, for he was feeling more hot and anxious than ever in his life before. *There were four animals in front of them!*

"Do you see, Piglet? Look at their tracks! Three, as it were, Woozles, and one, as it was, Wizzle. *Another Woozle has joined them!*"

And so it seemed to be. There were the tracks; crossing over each other here, getting muddled up with each other there; but, quite plainly every now and then, the tracks of four sets of paws.

"I *think,*" said Piglet, when he had licked the tip of his nose too, and found that it brought very little comfort, "I *think* that I have just remembered something that I forgot to do yesterday and shan't be able to do tomorrow. It's a very particular morning thing, that has to be done between the hours of—What would you say the time was?"

"About twelve," said Winnie-the-Pooh, looking at the sun.

"Between, as I was saying, the hours of twelve and twelve five. So, really, dear old Pooh, if you'll excuse me—*What's that?*"

Pooh looked up at the sky, and then, as he heard
the whistle again, he looked up into the branches of
a big oak-tree, and then he saw a friend of his.

"It's Christopher Robin," he said.

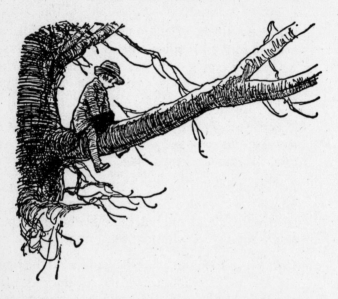

"Ah, then you'll be all right," said Piglet, and he
trotted off home as quickly as he could, very glad to
be Out of All Danger again.

"The Woozle Walk," Rabbit concluded. "A smashing exercise for our Club."

"Especially good for the Piglet Shape, and a Sizable Companion," said Piglet.

"Then you *like* the Woozle Walk, Piglet?" I asked.

"Now that it's over, I like it."

"It's educational," said Christopher Robin. "It teaches the difference between Woozles and Wizzles. And *I* get to climb a tree!"

"Why don't we all go climbing trees?" I suggested. "Then, maybe an hour of our stretch-and-flex drills, followed by—"

"Let's look for dragons!" said Christopher Robin. "There's a nest of them lurking down by the floody stream."

"**Dragon Hunting**," said Rabbit. "Another Forest Exercise. Exclusive. Natural. Impressive."

"This would be one of our best ones, Rabbit,"

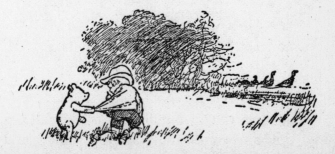

said Christopher Robin. "It begins with a march into Dragon Territory, with great caution. You head for the river, where the dragons cluster. As you near the water, you duck down low and listen for their characteristic noise."

"Dragons make noise?" asked Piglet.

"Can they run?" asked Pooh.

"They make a gabble noise," Christopher Robin told them. "It's like the cry of the Heffalump, only not so soggy."

"I'll wager they *do* run," said Piglet, getting behind Pooh.

"Then it gets Ferocious," Christopher Robin continued, "because you have to jump out and frighten the dragons." He turned to me. "A sudden noise tends to startle them, you know."

"No, I didn't."

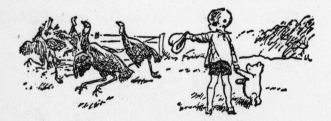

"And then you cry out, Shoo! And they all run away. Unless of course they saw you coming and didn't get startled."

"What would happen then?" Piglet worried.

"Well . . . They just might get Nosy."

"I don't like that exercise," said Piglet.

"That's all right," said Rabbit. "There are plenty of others."

"Yes," I agreed. "Planting Haycorns. Wind Walking. Jumping and—"

"I didn't mean those," said Rabbit.

"What's wrong with those?"

"They're not Friendly enough," said Pooh.

"What?" I cried out. "But I thought—"

"I'm sure they're all good in their way," Pooh added quickly, "and I don't at all mean to dislike them. It's just that they don't seem as Hummy as these others in Rabbit's Club."

"But Pooh, don't you want to become a Bear of Great Strength? And what about Going for the Hum?"

"No one," said Rabbit, "needs to teach Pooh anything about Hums."

"We were singing some just before," said Piglet.

"It's another Club Exercise."

"Everyone just stands around and sings?" I said. "That's another Club Exercise?"

'You can sit if you want," said Pooh. "You might come and join us tomorrow. We're going to sing after the Marathon."

"I'll handle this, Pooh," said Rabbit. "The Forest Exercise Club is holding its first race. We'll be running from Christopher Robin's the long way round the Hundred Acre Wood to Eeyore's. First one home is the winner. And that's the whole of it."

"Well, well, well."

"I have to arrange with Owl about the checkpoints," said Rabbit, scratching his whiskers pensively. "Carry on." And he joined Owl in The New Wolery.

"What sort of prize should the winner get tomorrow at the Marathon?" Christopher Robin wondered.

"Most people like a jar of hunny when they win a race," said Pooh.

"On the other hand," offered Piglet, "a balloon is often popular."

"I'll leave you to your planning," I sighed.

"Aren't you going to help us imagine some more exercises?"

"You don't need my help anymore, Piglet," I said sadly, as I started to leave.

"Please!"

"Just one more," said Christopher Robin. "With ever so many boxes and charts?"

"A special exercise just for us," urged Pooh. "And you could join in, too. It's our favorite! A new kind of frisk!"

I paused. "What is it called?"

"Silly Dancing!"

"Oh, good grief!"

"It's a frisk for *all* Shapes!"

"Not all Shapes, Pooh," said Piglet. "I couldn't see Owl doing it."

"Or Kanga," said Christopher Robin.

"Or most Wizzles."

"Well," said Pooh, "it's certainly good for the Pooh Shape."

"Couldn't you help us plan it?" asked Christopher Robin. "You might say it was to help celebrate our graduation."

"Well, all right," I said. "I guess an athlete should know how to lose gracefully. What's Silly Dancing?"

"I invented it," Christopher Robin began, "when I was running around a table one day."

"Why were you running around a table?"

"Just because."

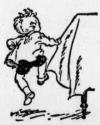
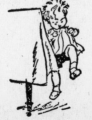
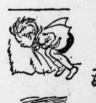

"Because it loosens up the bodily attach-
ments," Piglet suggested.

"It feels especially tickly," Pooh offered,
"about the knees."

"All right. What's the technique?"

"No technique," Christopher Robin answered
"You just get up and do it."

"Some can and some can't," said Pooh, I hope
with a kindly intention. "That's the way it is."

"Don't look at me," said Piglet. "I just do what
they do."

And all three of them got right up and did it.

From that session I gleaned the following
notes:

THE EXPERTS' CORNER:
ADVICE FROM NOTED ATHLETES
ON SILLY DANCING

CHRISTOPHER ROBIN:
The basic motion is a left-right, left-right of the
feet, pushing one's weight off the ground with vigorous toe placement and a sort of flying whoop in
the arms.

POOH:
A solid, unvaried up-and-down bounding works
well. Aim the head upward and keep the arms

rigid. The effect is that of a dense mound of India rubber dancing upon the earth. To avoid monotony, tour the site.

PIGLET:
Tiny leaps here and there, angled landings, and no sense of balance whatsoever are the theme of Piglet's style, though these sometimes lead to Falling Down, Bumping into Partners, and various other Failures of Amenity.

RECOMMENDED
DIRECTIONAL ADVANTAGES

PIGLET:	CHRISTOPHER ROBIN:	POOH:

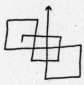

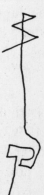

One difficulty many beginners face in undertaking Silly Dancing is its somewhat amorphous composition. "You just get up and do it" may be refreshingly simple after the many paragraphs of material one encounters in most workout manuals, yet it seems to lack something in instruction. However, as an eye-witness of Silly Dancing's three ranking experts getting up and doing it, I can vouch for the completeness of this instruction. You *do* just get up and do it.

However, as a supplement—and because Pooh, Piglet, and Christopher Robin were thrilled at the prospect of another box—I offer the box on the following page.

Watching Pooh, Piglet, and Christopher Robin at their favorite exercise, I had to admit that they did after all know better than I how to manage a workout. There was definitely something in Silly Dancing.

So I joined in. I flew with Christopher Robin and I bounded with Pooh and I leaped with Piglet; I posed "Cottleston Pie" riddles during the resting period; and then I got up again and danced myself silly. I don't know if it was actually good for my muscles, but it felt wonderful.

TYPICAL BEGINNER'S QUESTIONS
ABOUT SILLY DANCING

1. "Is it necessary or admirable to sing The Hums of Pooh while dancing?"

   ANSWER: It may be helpful, but it is not required. However, you may want to pose "Cottleston Pie" riddles during the resting periods.

2. "Then one should schedule resting periods?"

   ANSWER: If one wants to rest.

3. "What personal qualities contribute to a silly dance and which qualities hinder it?"

   ANSWER: Dignity, self-importance, ridigity of temperament, and an obsession about organization will neutralize the exuberance of the exercise. Friendliness will exhilarate it.

4. "Isn't Silly Dancing like Jumping and Squeaking?"

   ANSWER: That depends on how you dance and whether or not you squeak.

5. "What if how I dance is jumping and I *do* squeak?"

   ANSWER: Then, yes, Silly Dancing is like Jumping and Squeaking. But that's your fault, isn't it?

II. THE FOREST
MARATHON

Rabbit was in his element on the day of the Marathon—*his* Marathon, really. For one thing, virtually everyone of note had entered, even Owl, who was planning to fly the course, by special dispensation of Christopher Robin and the realization that the Owl Shape just doesn't navigate land at any speed to speak of.

I volunteered to help Rabbit man the checkpoints, but he insisted on handling it himself, as he was the fastest runner in the Forest. Anyway, it was Rabbit's Marathon, not mine.

Marathon excitement resounded through the Forest from Galleons Lap to the Poohsticks Bridge. Rabbit set the tempo with crisp Organization. Roo and Tigger were unspeakably thrilled; they bounced each other at least seven times, more or less accidentally, to Kanga's refrain of "Now Tigger, you must be more careful!" And Rabbit's friends and relations were so Expectant and Awed that it might have been the North Pole Expedition all over again.

"There you are, Piglet," said Rabbit, checking him off on his clipboard as he trudged warily up the hill. "You're number seventeen, then."

"Seventeen?" Piglet echoed. "How many are there in this race?"

"Seven. Why?"

"Why am I number seventeen?"

"Because you are," Rabbit explained. "Here's Owl."

"On such a fine day as this," said Owl, "my second cousin Gervase become Giddy with Flight, crashed headlong into a birch tree, and broke—"

"Owl!" cried Roo. "Are you in the race, too? Because I am. So's Tigger. I'm number six and Tigger's fourteen. What's your number, Owl?"

"Now Roo, dear," said Kanga. "Why don't you come over here and show Christopher Robin your starting position?"

"Rabbit, does Owl have a number? What number will Pooh have? Hullo, Piglet! I'm number six!"

"As I was saying, my cousin Gervase broke his—"

"Tigger, what's your number? Oh yes, you're

fourteen. And I'm *six!*"

"He crashed so badly that he utterly broke—"

"I like being six. Rabbit, could I be seven, too?"

"Roo, dear—"

"Cousin Gervase—"

"It's as usual, I see. Larking About. Pointless Exclamations. And Intense Crowding Among the Bystanders."

Eeyore had arrived.

"Eeyore," said Rabbit, checking him off on his sheet, "you're number twenty-four."

"Is that the worst number? The one nobody else wanted?"

"It's just a number."

"That's right. Let's give Eeyore the dull number. The one without a square root. Any number at all, that's Eeyore's."

"And here's Pooh. Now we can start."

"Bear!"

"Pooh, what number are you? I'm six and Tigger's—"

"Actually, cousin Gervase not only broke his—"

"Roo, dear—"

Christopher Robin hugged Pooh, Rabbit assigned him a number, Piglet was found to have disappeared, I went into Christopher Robin's house to get Piglet, Piglet explained that he had just gone in to count balloons for the Party After, Owl finally got it out (to Kanga, who wasn't listening because she was keeping an eye on Roo) that what his second cousin Gervase broke was his crown, Roo (who *had* been listening) asked if Owl's second cousin Gervase was a king . . . and Rabbit called everyone to the starting line.

Christopher Robin had a red flag.

"Now remember, everyone," Rabbit warned, "you must pass each of the three checkpoints. First, the Bee Tree. Next, the Six Pine Trees. Third, the Woozle Spinney. And fourth is home, Eeyore's place. The first one there wins."

Rabbit's friends and relations cheered.

"None of that, now. Save it for the winner. Any questions?"

"I have one," said Eeyore. "Would it be at all possible to ask Tigger to stand off a bit instead of treading on my feet?"

"Spread out, fellows," said Rabbit.

"Sorry to be a bother," said Eeyore. "It's just that feet come in handy sometimes."

"If there are no further questions—"

"None," said Eeyore. "Except that one of the spectators is making a rude noise. If you can't keep your own family in line, Rabbit, what are the rest of us to think, I ask you?"

"Never mind," said Rabbit. "Christopher Robin."

Christopher Robin stepped forward. "I'll say

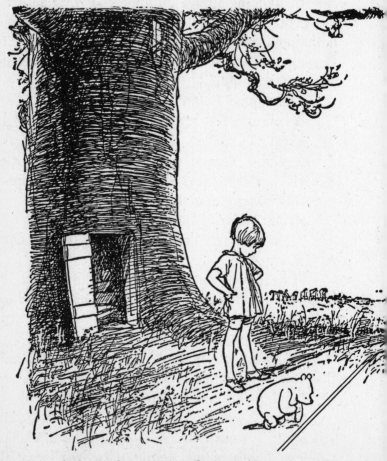

*Pooh takes his position at the starting line
as Rabbit musters the other runners.*

Take your marks, then Get set, then Run! And I'll drop the flag. When I drop the flag—"

"Everybody runs!" cried Roo.

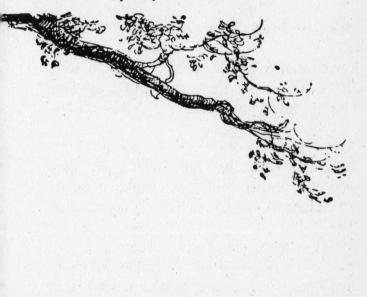

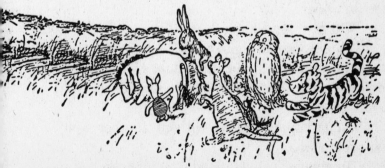

Rabbit's friends and relations cheered.

"Let's run *now!*" shouted Tigger.

"Not yet," said Rabbit. "Christopher Robin will tell when it's time."

"It's time," said Christopher Robin. "On your marks!"

Kanga leaned into a crouch. Eeyore braced himself. Pooh flexed his Shape and Got Ready. Tigger bounced about in a frenzy. Piglet smelled a daisy.

"Get set!"

"We're *off!*" screamed Roo, and Tigger, overwhelmed with anticipation, took off like a comet.

"Wait for me, Tigger!" squeaked Roo, running after him.

Rabbit's friends and relations cheered.

"Roo dear," Kanga began—but Roo was chasing after Tigger and calling for him to wait, and couldn't hear.

"Oh my," said Kanga.

"Ought we call them back?" asked Owl.

"They're already in the distance," said Christopher Robin. "Maybe everyone should just start running now."

Kanga bounced away without another word, her eye on Roo.

"In my day," Owl opined, "mature sportsmanship was the mark of the true athlete. Enthusiasm

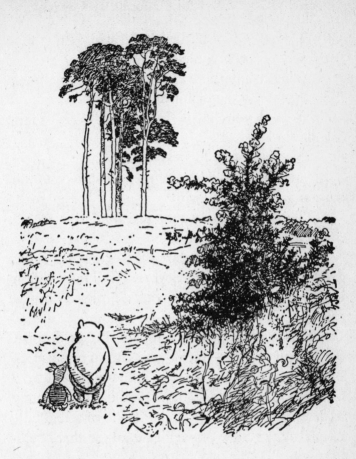

has its place, yes, but—"

"Come on, Piglet," said Pooh. "The race has begun."

Side by side, Piglet and Pooh began to walk toward the first checkpoint. I followed and walked along beside them as Owl flew past us overhead.

"Excuse me for butting in," I said. "But you're supposed to run in a race."

"This is only the warmup part," Pooh replied. "We'll probably run later on."

"Would you like to come with us?" Piglet asked.

"No, I'll catch up to you later."

Back at the starting line, Eeyore was still braced and ready to go.

"The race has begun, Eeyore," Rabbit was saying. "Everyone has left."

"The race doesn't start till Christopher Robin drops the red flag," said Eeyore. "Call me old-fashioned, but when I play a game I play it by the rules."

Thus instructed, Christopher Robin dropped the flag and Eeyore trotted off. After a few feet, he stopped, turned, and asked, "Is there to be a prize for the winner? I realize that even if I should come in first, someone will probably think of a reason to disqualify me. Still, I thought I'd ask, so that in case I do win, I'll know what I didn't get."

"The prize is my alphabet book," said Christopher Robin. "And you'll have it if you win, no matter what anyone says."

"Christopher Robin's alphabet book!" Eeyore repeated, as he started off again. "How sad I'll be when I don't get it!"

"I'll get off to the first checkpoint," said Rabbit.

"I'll start getting the party ready, and wrap up my alphabet book," said Christopher Robin. "Are you coming?"

"I don't know," I said. "I think I'll take a leisurely walk through the Forest. Maybe I'll see you later and maybe I won't."

"It would help," Rabbit began. "Mind you, I don't say that it's necessary, but it would *help* if you were to drop in at the second checkpoint so I could go right from the Bee Tree to Eeyore's. What I mean is, it would save time."

He's got some nerve, I thought, asking me to help out in an event that was designed to make me look Unnecessary in the Forest. "I might," I said.

Rabbit sped off, Christopher Robin went inside to see about the party things, and I breezed through the center of the Forest, listening to those wonderful noises that somehow seem most vivid not when you arrive but when you are about to leave. I made it a nice long walk.

As I reached the Pine Trees, I heard voices calmly discussing the advantages of the various Shapes in running away from Enraged Woozles.

"The Tigger Shape would run faster," Piglet was saying.

"Yes. But the Tigger Shape would be Noticeable," Pooh answered. "The Piglet Shape could hide."

"What about the Pooh Shape, Pooh?"

After a pause, he said, "I would be somewhere else at that time."

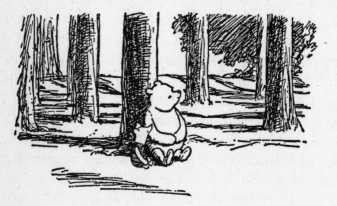

"Somewhere else is right," I put in, coming up to them. "Here you are, sitting around and chatting right in the middle of a race. Kanga, Tigger, and Roo must be nearly to the finish by now."

"No, they went home," said Piglet.

"*What?*"

"Roo got hiccoughs and Tigger got hungry, so Kanga took them home till it's time for the party. They were passing by their house, anyway."

Just then Eeyore loped past us.

"That's right," he said. "Don't say hallo. It's only Eeyore."

Whereupon we all did cry out hallo.

"There must be someone important behind me," said Eeyore, trotting along into the trees.

"Well, at least Eeyore's still in the race," I said. "Are you?"

"Of course we are," said Piglet. "We may not finish it today, that's all."

"We're inventing a new exercise," said Pooh. "**Race Resting**."

"Oh, please."

"Race Resting is more satisfying than plain resting," Piglet told me. It's especially Friendly to sit and look at the trees when others are running around and such."

"If only we'd thought to bring along a snack," said Pooh.

"Why don't we get one now?"

"Yes, let's."

"Pooh," I called out, "aren't you forgetting about Calories?"

"I thought we were allowed an extra smackerel or two if we're running," he said, turning back.

"Pooh, you aren't running."

"Will we see you at the party?" Piglet asked me.

"Aren't you going to finish the race?"

"Of course we are. Maybe not today, though."

It looked like Rabbit's Marathon would not go off *quite* as smoothly as he had planned. Suddenly I decided to join him at the finish line to see the fun, and jogged toward the Hundred Acre Wood, where I met up with Owl, obviously heading for Christopher Robin's.

"Giving up, Owl?"

"It appears that the Wind Longitude is somewhat less than Conducive."

"I'll bet the Latitude's pretty heavy too, eh, Owl?"

"Ah, yes, that may well be." He looked at me the way the others usually look at him, spread his wings, and—Longitude and Latitude notwithstanding—took off for Christopher Robin's without another word.

Cutting through the Hundred Acre Wood, I found Rabbit all alone at Eeyore's, his whiskers twitching with disapproval.

"Well?" I said as I came up.

"Something's wrong," Rabbit noticed. "No one has come in yet. They should all have finished by now."

"Owl gave up. I think his wings were tired."

"That's all right. It's Tigger or Kanga, I expect. One or the other."

"They gave up, too. Roo had to be taken home."

Rabbit took this bravely. "It will look odd that Pooh or Piglet should win. It can't be helped, but it will look odd."

"Pooh and Piglet went home for a snack," I said. "They'll just continue on to the party. Looks like the Forest Exercise Club is getting off to a problematic start, eh what?"

"I see something!" he cried, hopefully. "Something is coming through the trees. From the third checkpoint."

Sure enough, something *was* coming toward us from the distance—very slowly.

"I can't make out who it is," I said. "But I suppose it must be Eeyore. He's the only one left."

"Eeyore," said Rabbit, almost plaintively. "It *ought* to have been Tigger or Kanga."

It took quite some time for Eeyore to arrive. He was barely strolling, head down and eyes half shut, and he seemed singularly unimpressed when Rabbit greeted him with a hearty Hallo.

"You've won, Eeyore," Rabbit announced. "You've won the Forest Marathon!"

"No, I didn't," said Eeyore. "Somebody else will have to win."

"But you came in first, Eeyore," I said. "You ran the course and crossed the finishing line."

"What finishing line?"

"This is the finishing line," said Rabbit. "Right here."

"This is also where I happen to live. That's the reason I'm here. I stopped racing a long time ago and I just took the shortest way home. It's not my fault if you want to mark off sections of the Forest for idle amusement."

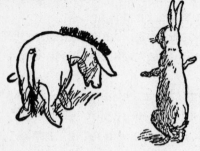

"Eeyore, you came here," Rabbit persisted. "It doesn't matter *why!* You came here, and this is where you win, so you're the winner!"

"*I'll* decide whether I won or not," Eeyore replied. "Now, if you don't mind, I'd like to be alone. It's very disheartening to lose a race, and I don't want company just now."

"What's taking everyone so long?" asked Christopher Robin, coming up with his alphabet book. "The party's all ready."

"Losing a race and not being invited to a party, all at once," said Eeyore. "This is certainly a big day for me."

"Eeyore refused to win," I said.

"He came in first," Rabbit explained. "But now he says he wasn't in the race."

"Of course he was," said Christopher Robin. "I started him off myself. And here's the alphabet book. Don't you want it?"

Eeyore sighed, looked at the book, and sighed again. Christopher Robin opened it and turned some of the pages so Eeyore could see.

"Christopher Robin's alphabet book," said Eeyore quietly.

"With color," said Christopher Robin. "See?"

"What's that?" asked Eeyore, pointing to something.

"That's the letter D."

"And what is that a picture of, there on the same page as D?"

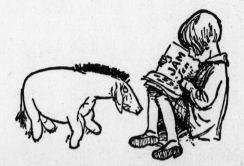

"Why, that's you, Eeyore!" cried Christopher Robin.

Eeyore suppressed a thrill. "D is for Eeyore?" he asked.

"Well, no . . . but it comes down to being the same thing."

"My, my," said Eeyore. "I'm in Christopher Robin's alphabet book."

"Hallo!" cried Pooh and Piglet, coming down from Christopher Robin's.

"Eeyore won the Marathon!" said Christopher Robin.

"The party's already begun," said Piglet. "Tigger has started on the cake."

"We'd better get back," said Christopher Robin. "Come along, everyone."

"Pooh," said Eeyore as we started up, "do you know who's in Christopher Robin's alphabet book?"

"I am," said Pooh.

"You are?"

"The letter B is for Bear," Christopher Robin announced.

"Is Rabbit in this book, too?" Eeyore asked.

"No. R is for rain. There's a picture of some, raining."

Rabbit led the way with Christopher Robin, followed by Pooh and Piglet. Eeyore and I, carrying

Eeyore's prize, brought up the rear.

"I don't mind that Pooh is in the book," Eeyore told me confidentially as we walked. "But I shouldn't have liked it if Rabbit was in it as well. Do you see what I mean?"

"Yes, Eeyore. I believe I do."

12. AN EXERCISE
FOR RESTING UP AFTER

It was generally agreed that the party after the Marathon was the best party anyone could remember. Owl delivered several speeches, Rabbit let Roo show him how to frisk, and Eeyore complained about Tigger only three or four times at most.

"What I would like," said Christopher Robin, as he, Pooh, Piglet, and I were clearing up after the party, "is one for Pooh and Piglet and me."

"One what?"

"An exercise, of course! But a very quiet one. Something without balloons and pots and things. Something for when we're having our picnics at the top of the Forest. A quiet, sharing sort of exercise."

"A tidy one," said Piglet. "Something smallish that doesn't bump about quite so much as the others do. But then," he added sadly, "I don't imagine it would be an exercise anymore."

"You mean," I said, "something for when you've just eaten and everyone is sitting back or lying down, talking about when you last saw the King of Belgium?"

"Yes," said Christopher Robin. "When no one knows where you are except the grass and the trees, and they won't tell."

"Yes," said Pooh. "That time."

"Just that time," said Piglet.

"There's a special exercise that you could do then that no one else in the Forest can: **Listening to the Sky**.

"Why can't the others do that?" asked Pooh.

"Because this exercise calls for sensitivity, for taking in what goes on around you. It's almost as if you were watching the world do *its* exercises, and that takes a certain sense of the world that the others don't have. Rabbit is too busy and Tigger too bouncy. Kanga always has her eye on Roo. Owl doesn't listen and Eeyore only hears thunderclouds."

"Is that what it is?" Piglet asked. "Listening to the sky?"

"Sensitivity can take that form."

"And *we* can do that?" said Pooh. "By ourselves, quietly together?"

"We just lie there and listen?" Piglet asked "We don't move at *all?*"

"That's right."

He seemed doubtful. "This is the first time I've ever heard of a lazy exercise. What part of the body is it good for?"

"The soul. Your imagination needs a little workout every now and then too, you know."

"I like it," said Christopher Robin. "But what are we supposed to hear the sky say?"

"I can't tell you that. It's different each time and for each person. Everyone hears something else."

They thought this over for a bit. Then Christopher Robin said, "Let's go on a picnic, and try out our new exercise."

"It isn't new," I told him. "You've been doing it all your life. You just didn't have a name for it."

"It sounds like doing Nothing," said Christopher Robin.

"That's just what it is."

"How do you do Nothing?" asked Pooh, after he had wondered for a long time.

"Well, it's when people call out at you just as you're going off to do it, What are you going to do, Christopher Robin, and you say, Oh, nothing, and then you go and do it."

"Oh, I see," said Pooh.

"This is a nothing sort of thing that we're doing now."

"Oh, I see," said Pooh again.

"It means just going along, listening to all the things you can't hear, and not bothering."

"Oh!" said Pooh.

They walked on, thinking of This and That, and by-and-by they came to an enchanted place on the very top of the Forest called Galleons Lap, which is sixty-something trees in a circle; and Christopher Robin knew that it was enchanted because nobody had ever been able to count whether it was sixty-three or sixty-four, not even when he tied a piece of string round each tree after he had counted it. Being enchanted, its floor was not like the floor of the Forest, gorse and bracken and heather, but close-set grass, quiet and smooth and green. It was the only place in the Forest where you could sit down carelessly, without getting up again almost at once and looking for somewhere else. Sitting there they could see the whole world spread out until it reached the sky, and whatever there was all the world over was with them in Galleons Lap.

"Why is it that you are recommending an exercise like this?" asked Piglet. "I thought you only liked the bouncy ones."

"I guess I'm finally trying to see things your

way, Piglet."

"Come on, Bear," said Christopher Robin.

"The best thing about it," said Pooh, "is that instead of having to go home after the party with all the fun suddenly over, *we* get to start another party. I like that."

"Coming?" Christopher Robin asked me.

"Not this time."

As they headed off to Galleons Lap, I stood very still where I was, and I, too, listened: to the whispers and song of an Enchanted Place, one that will stay Enchanted, I had come to realize, no matter what wind blows in from other, less enchanted, places.

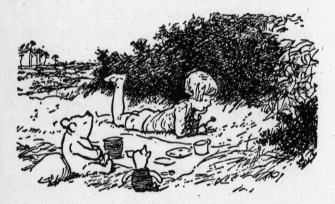